Basic Management for
Staff Nurses

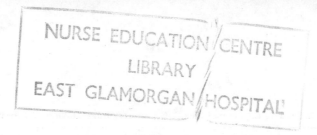
Basic Management for Staff Nurses

Edited by

Nancy MacLeod Nicol RGN, ONC, RCT, RNT, *Senior Tutor, Continuing Education Department, Lothian College of Nursing and Midwifery, South Division, Edinburgh*
and
Stanley Walker RGN, RCNT, RNT, STD, *Director of Nurse Education, Lothian College of Nursing and Midwifery, South Division, Edinburgh*

CHAPMAN & HALL
London · Glasgow · New York · Tokyo · Melbourne · Madras

Published by Chapman & Hall, 2-6 Boundary Row, London SE1 8HN

Chapman & Hall, 2-6 Boundary Row, London SE1 8HN, UK

Blackie Academic & Professional, Wester Cleddens Road,
Bishopbriggs, Glasgow G64 2NZ, UK

Chapman & Hall, 29 West 35th Street, New York NY10001, USA

Chapman & Hall Japan, Thomson Publishing Japan, Hirakawacho
Nemoto Building, 6F, 1-7-11 Hirakawa-cho, Chiyoda-ku, Tokyo 102,
Japan

Chapman & Hall Australia, Thomas Nelson Australia, 102 Dodds
Street, South Melbourne, Victoria 3205, Australia

Chapman & Hall India, R. Seshadri, 32 Second Main Road, CIT East,
Madras 600 035, India

First edition 1991
Reprinted 1993

© 1991 N. MacLeod and S. Walker

Typeset in 10/12pt Palatino by Input Typesetting Ltd, London
Printed in Great Britain by The Ipswich Book Co., Ipswich

ISBN 0 412 35520 5

A catalogue record for this book is available from the British Library
Library of Congress Cataloging-in-Publication Data available

Contents

Contributors

Pauline Baber,
BEd, RGN, RM, RCNT, RNT,
Senior Tutor, Lothian College of Nursing and Midwifery, South Division

Bill Beaton,
BSC (Hons), DN, RGN, RMNH, RNT,
Nurse Teacher, Lothian College of Nursing and Midwifery, South Division

Nicola Downing,
MA, MSc (Nursing Education), RGN, RNT,
Nurse Teacher, Lothian College of Nursing and Midwifery, South Division

Rose Fleming,
Diploma in Management (Nursing Administration), RGN, RM,
Manager, Area Sterilising Centre, Lothian Health Board

Nancy MacLeod Nicol,
RGN, ONC, RCNT, RNT
Senior Tutor, Lothian College of Nursing and Midwifery, South Division

Dirjodhun Mojee,
BSc (Social Sciences), MSc (Nursing Education), RGN, ONC
Nurse Teacher, Lothian College of Nursing and Midwifery, South Division

Jim Reid,
RGN, RMN, RNT,
Nurse Teacher, Lothian College of Nursing and Midwifery, South Division

Arthur Thwaites,
RGN, RMN, Tropical Nursing Certificate,
Nursing Officer (retired), Lothian Health Board

Stanley Walker, RGN, RCNT, RNT, STD
Director of Nurse Education, Lothian
College of Nursing and Midwifery,
South Division

Acknowledgements

The preparation of this book involved much time and work from the willing group of contributors. We would like to thank them all for meeting the deadlines and producing such good chapters.

However, this book would never have come to fruition had it not been for the many staff nurses who have attended courses in the Continuing Education Department over the years, and who have encouraged us in our work to help make them the backbone of the nursing profession now and in the future.

Finally our thanks to secretaries, librarians, colleagues and friends who willingly typed manuscripts, challenged our opinions, proof-read the scripts and encouraged us towards publication.

Preface

This book is for all staff nurses, particularly the newly qualified and those who have returned to nursing after a break in service, but we hope it will also be helpful to enrolled nurses and final year student nurses.

All of the authors are involved in teaching staff nurses on courses immediately after their registration, and were concerned with the lack of basic readable literature available for course participants, and for those staff nurses who worked in areas where no such courses were being held.

A job description may give a staff nurse an insight into what is involved in the post of staff nurse, but sound knowledge, skill and experience are required for fulfilment of the post. This book, whilst not a textbook, should meet the needs of the former.

The structure of the National Health Service varies in the four parts of the United Kingdom, and we have tried to cover the differences so as not to have it read too parochially.

As nursing is still a predominantly female profession, the pronoun she is used throughout to refer to the nurse whilst the pronoun he, to the patient. This is in no way intended to slight the many worthy male nurses or female patients!

Nancy MacLeod Nicol

Foreword

It is in the nature of things that by far the greatest number of trained nurses involved in direct patient care are of the grades of staff nurse and for that reason alone this book is a must. The book has been written with a profound awareness of what the newly qualified staff nurse or those returning after a break in service will need to know to enable them, with confidence, to put into practice the knowledge and skills, taught, learnt and practised during training. It is immensely readable. Anyone who dips into its pages will want to read on. They are full of interest; a mass of facts, plainly set out with humorous illustrations to drive the point home.

In periods of great change – which is an ongoing state within the National Health Service – the nursing profession cannot escape the inevitable consequences that such a world of change brings about. A service which is completely dependent on the quality and expertise of its personnel needs to establish fundamental principles of continuing education and training. We know to our cost that inadequate preparation threatens the overall effectiveness of our profession and ultimately the patient.

The importance of continuing education for the newly qualified staff nurse, although embraced in principle by the profession, is not always put into practice. For this reason, if for no other, the profession owes a debt to the authors of this book who have extended to the reader through this book their own composite skills and experience.

To those like me who have had the privilege of reading this book, I would emphasise our professional responsibility and commitment to ensure that it is read by all trained nurses.

Isabel G. Duncan
Secretary, Scottish Board
Royal College of Nursing

1

Professional development

Stanley Walker

1.1. Introduction

Professional development from the point of registration is essential
to ensure the highest quality of care, and in this context, the
American Nurses' Association (1975) definition is particularly
appropriate.

> Continuing education in nursing consists of planned learning
> experiences beyond a basic nursing education programme.
> These experiences are designed to promote the development of
> knowledge, skills and attitudes for the enhancement of nursing
> practice, thus improving health care to the public.

When considering your professional development it is essential
to establish at the outset the following three key factors.

1. As a Registered Nurse you are obliged under the United Kingdom Central Council Code of Professional Conduct (1984) to
   ensure that you 'take every reasonable opportunity to maintain
   and improve professional knowledge and competence'.
2. Your career prospects will depend on how you manage your
   professional development.
3. You, and you alone, are accountable for your professional
   development.

So not only are you obliged to ensure that you advance your
professional knowledge, but clearly the process involves commitment and motivation on the part of the individual. So, where and
when do you begin?
Clearly you begin when you qualify as a registered nurse. Where
you begin will demand your thought, consideration and perhaps
the advice of others.
Before you decide on a plan of action, you may find it helpful

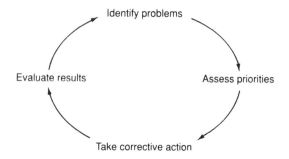

Figure 1.1 The problem-solving cycle

to carry out a self-assessment to identify priorities in planning your career development.

In assessing yourself it is useful to examine how effective you are in your present post, as this will enable you to identify areas in which you could improve your performance.

In determining how effective you are you will find it useful to ask yourself a number of questions:

1. Are there any aspects of your work you like better than others, and why?
2. Are there any aspects of your work you dislike, and why?
3. Are there any aspects of your work you find difficult, and why?
4. Do you feel that your capabilities are fully utilized?
5. Can you make any changes which will increase your effectiveness?
6. Could any additional experience or training improve your performance?

The answers to these questions should enable you to identify your priorities in dealing with short-term career development, and should be discussed with your immediate superior.

Having identified your priorities use the method outlined in Figure 1.1 for dealing with each item on your list.

By repeating the process your list of problems will decrease until they have all been resolved.

There is evidence to suggest that individuals are motivated by achieving short-term goals which lead to early success, and therefore it is important that employee and employer should capitalize on this to ensure short-term career development deals with the individual's immediate work problems.

The progress you make will be largely dependent on your degree of motivation. To succeed you must be committed to a course of action which may require you to curtail other interests for a period of time.

In considering your commitment you must identify how practical your course of action will be, given your other family and personal commitments. How much time can you put aside each day for studying? Does it fit in with your work schedule? Or will your employer be flexible and allow you to have time off or special shift patterns? Is there a financial commitment? If so, how much will it cost and can you afford it, and will your employer help with the cost?

It is important to discuss your intentions with your employer to ensure that there is mutual commitment to your course of action. This should be explored well in advance to enable you to meet any deadlines such as application for places on courses, study leave, special off duty and financial assistance.

Having considered some general points on career development, let's consider some approaches in identifying career pathways.

Whatever you choose should be compatible with your professional interests, your personal skills and academic ability, and may be influenced by advice and appraisal from your employer. The professional pathway approach is usually defined by an interest in a particular clinical field, but this may change from time to time or diversify into a speciality within a specific area of interest.

In most instances this will require a post-registration course, and care must be exercised to ensure that the course is recognized by the National Board of the country in which it is taken.

Always obtain a copy of the course curriculum, as courses of a similar nature will vary in content depending on the clinical experience available.

Find out from your employer whether you could be seconded on full salary to undertake the course; alternatively, you may wish to apply as an independent candidate. Remember that if you are seconded you may be required to give a commitment to your employers to remain in their employment for a period of time after the course.

Most post-registration courses are over-subscribed, so ensure that you apply well in advance of the time you hope to commence. Details of where courses are offered can be obtained through the respective National Boards in each country of the United Kingdom.

Career pathways which develop existing personal qualities and skill are most likely to give the greatest job satisfaction, and will therefore be significant in deciding future career prospects and promotion. In this category you should consider areas of work in which you feel comfortable and confident. These may be in teaching, counselling, managing and controlling staff, or research. Any of these areas can be developed either through in-service study days, by attending conferences, or through more formal courses.

Academic ability is an area which concerns most individuals when considering further education and nurses are no exception to the norm. It is of interest to note that many nurses who trained through conventional courses in schools and colleges of nursing go on to achieve graduate qualifications, and indeed some have graduated to PhD level. Most individuals tend to underestimate their capabilities, and it is always useful to discuss your ability to succeed in advanced study with a senior colleague or academic who should be able to give advice on the academic level of an advanced course of study.

If you still have doubts then it may be sensible to try a short Open University course or an A level course to see how you cope with in-depth study.

Having considered your career development under these three areas you need now to formulate a plan of action which will identify short and long-term goals.

Try working out a realistic timescale, say over a period of at least six years. This period of time has been chosen as most nurses achieve charge nurse grade during it, and, therefore, your plan of action should aim at achieving promotion to this level.

Next, identify what courses of study are necessary to enable you to achieve your goal and decide when and where you will make application.

Opportunities for study leave and financial assistance need to be explored before you make formal application, and again this will require discussion with your superior.

Obtaining either of these may prove to be difficult, particularly the latter, so you may have to consider other sources which may offer you financial support.

Most Health Authorities allocate part of their budget for continuing education and your personnel officer should be able to advise on this matter.

Courses leading to teaching qualifications in nursing are sponsored by the National Boards and advice can be obtained through a Director or Principal of a College of Nursing.

Finally your hospital may have specific endowments which have been bequeathed for educational studies for qualified nurses, and your Director of Nursing Services or General Manager should be able to advise you on these.

What courses of study are available? The difficulty which faces most nurses is obtaining information on what is available and in this part of the chapter we shall identify some of the range and types of courses available and suitable for nurses at Staff Nurse grade.

1.2. Clinical courses

England

The English National Board approves a wide range of courses which can last from 8 to 72 weeks, leading, depending on the course taken, either to a certificate or to a statement of attendance. Details of all ENB Courses are available in the ENB booklet *Notes on the outline curricula* (1987).

Scotland

The National Board for Scotland approves a range of clinical Modules leading to a Diploma in Professional Studies. Three Modules are required in Professional Studies I, and three in Professional Studies II to successfully complete the Diploma.

Wales

The Welsh National Board is developing a new pattern of courses in professional practice leading to a Certificate in Professional Practice. The Certificate is awarded after completion of one common core module and two clinical modules.

Northern Ireland

The National Board for Northern Ireland is currently revising and developing a new scheme of continuing education.

Midwifery Courses
are approved by all National Boards in The United Kingdom.

1.3. Non-clinical courses

These are available on the following topics.

1. Assessing and examining learners
2. Counselling
3. Research
4. Industrial relations
5. Quality assurance

These lists are not exhaustive, but indicate some of the courses which are available. Local information on available courses can be obtained from the Principal or Director of Nurse Education at your nearest college or school of nursing, and National Boards will be able to advise on the complete list of courses available in each country of the United Kingdom.

1.4. Courses at Diploma/Degree level

Opportunities for nurses to study at Diploma or Degree level have increased during the last decade, and more recently the opportunity to study at this level on a part-time basis or by distance learning has also increased.

Information on available courses can be obtained from a College of Nursing or from Universities, Polytechnics or Colleges of Higher Education.

1.5. Teaching courses

Guidelines for entry requirements to teaching courses are specified by the United Kingdom Central Council, and can be obtained from the respective National Boards.

The guidelines specify the type and amount of post-registration experience required, and nurses considering a career in Nurse Education should obtain this information from their National Board. In addition it is useful to discuss your interest in education with the Principal or Director of Nurse Education in your area. A useful reference book which covers most professional courses available in The United Kingdom is *The Directory of Continuing*

Education and Training for Nurses, which should be available in all College of Nursing Libraries.

1.6. Distance learning

Difficulties in being released from duty and irregular working hours can present problems for many nurses who wish to undertake courses in professional development. Distance learning is an alternative to courses requiring regular attendance and makes education more accessible as well as being cost-effective. Like the Open University, distance learning centres provide the student with learning materials and access to a tutor counsellor usually attached to a local study centre.

Apart from the Open University, there are three other centres which provide distance learning courses suitable for nurses.

Distance Learning Centre
Polytechnic of the South Bank
PO Box 310
LONDON
SW4 9RZ

Barnet College
26 Danbury Street
LONDON
N1 8JU

Central Manchester College
Openshaw Centre
MANCHESTER
M11 2WH

1.7. Opportunities in the Armed Forces

Each of the three Armed Forces has a nursing branch, which offers short and long-term commissioned or non-commissioned service. Information on career opportunities and professional development in the Armed Forces can be obtained from Career Information Offices.

1.8. Working overseas

Many nurses take the opportunity to nurse overseas. Nursing in another country can be a useful and rewarding learning experience, and may offer you opportunities not available in this country to broaden and enhance your nursing skills.

For some nurses, the experience may not be so successful and you should ensure that you have considered all the facts before committing yourself to a contract of employment. You should find out as much as you can about the country, the hospital where you will be employed and, most importantly, the terms of your contract. You should also consider the culture of the country, and whether you feel you can adapt to any restraints which the culture may impose upon you.

If applying through an agency, ask to be put in contact with someone already nursing in the hospital. Find out whether you need reciprocal registration and whether you will be required to take an examination to enable you to register and practice in the country of employment.

The Royal College of Nursing has an International Department which can advise you about nursing in most overseas countries.

As well as International Nursing Agencies, you can apply for voluntary work overseas with Voluntary Services Overseas.

1.9. Other professional development activities

So far this chapter has concentrated on identifying priorities, planning personal development and has mentioned some of the possibilities which are available for professional development.

In looking at the wider aspects of career development it is worthwhile considering activities which can be undertaken on an individual basis and can be an advantage in promoting future career prospects. Such activities could include publishing articles in journals or carrying out small-scale research projects.

In addition it is possible to obtain scholarships from various foundations or awards to study a specific interest in a practical field of nursing, and you may find it useful to refer to the *Directory of Grant-Making Trusts*, the Royal College of Nursing and the Royal College of Midwives.

In reading this chapter you should now be aware that your initial nursing qualification is the foundation stone from which your career can develop. Professional development of the individual nurse is a joint responsibility shared by the Nurse Manager and the individual, but you should always remember that, as well as being accountable for the care you give to your patients, so too are you accountable to yourself for your own professional development.

1.10. Useful addresses

The English National Board for Nursing, Midwifery and Health Visiting
Victory House
170 Tottenham Court Road
LONDON
W1P 0HA

The National Board for Nursing, Midwifery and Health Visiting for Northern Ireland
RAC House
79 Chichester Street
BELFAST
BT1 4JE

Welsh National Board for Nursing, Midwifery and Health Visiting
Pearl Assurance House
Greyfriars Road
CARDIFF
CF1 3JN

The National Board for Nursing, Midwifery and Health Visiting for Scotland
22 Queen Street
EDINBURGH
EH2 1JX

The United Kingdom Central Council for Nursing, Midwifery and Health Visiting
23 Portland Place
LONDON
W1N 3AH

Voluntary Services Overseas
9 Belgrave Square
LONDON
SW1X 8PW

The Open University
PO Box 188
MILTON KEYNES
MK3 6HW

Royal College of Nursing
20 Cavendish Square
LONDON
W1M 0AB

Royal College of Midwives
15 Mansfield Street
LONDON
W1M 0BE

References

United Kingdom Central Council for Nursing, Midwifery and Health
    Visiting, (1984) *Code of Professional Conduct*, London.
English National Board (1987) Notes On The Outline Curricula (Booklet),
    London.

2

Communication

Bill Beaton

2.1. Introduction

'Communication forms the foundations of all nursing care, and yet strangely it is an area of nursing which has often been taken for granted or underestimated.'

Clarke, C. in Faulkner (1984)

The language of communication can seem complex and confusing. Such terms as interpersonal relationships, interpersonal communications, interpersonal skills, interpersonal relations, social skills and human skills are often encountered with little or no attempt made to explain them. For the purposes of this chapter such terms will be taken to be an integral part of communication itself.

It is expected that all trained nurses will be aware of the central importance of communication to all aspects of nursing care. Yet to judge by the volume of recent research on this subject, Kagan (1985) and Faulkner (1984) for example, it would appear that many nurses find it difficult to communicate effectively with both patients and colleagues.

Many reasons have been suggested to explain this situation. Among them are that nurses, perhaps, do not communicate effectively because they cannot cope with the stress of nursing. Or that nurses find undertaking physical tasks easier than having to talk to patients. Or that because nurses are worried about not having sufficient knowledge regarding a patient or his condition, they may be evasive and so ineffective communication may result. It is also suggested that nurses fail to communicate effectively because it is a subject which is neglected in basic training; that when it is taught, it is not properly assessed; and that as a result, nurses are left to learn from inappropriate role models, namely nurses, who themselves may not be well versed in communication (Maguire, P. in Kagan (1985)).

The nature of communication failures in nursing or their precise cause is not the main focus of this chapter. While accepting that

11

there are sometimes failures in communications, possibly for a number of different reasons, it is the purpose of this chapter to help the staff nurse to a greater understanding of the subject of communication and so to become herself a better communicator.

2.2. The paradox of communication

'It is clear though, . . . that the deficiencies in interpersonal skills use amongst nurses are great enough and important enough to patient care, to warrant immediate attention.'

Maguire, P. in Kagan (1985)

Consider a dictionary definition of communication, namely, 'impart, transmit, share' (Concise OED) and a common model of communication which states that for communication to take place, there will be a sender, a message and a receiver. In this model and definition, it would appear at first glance that to communicate is a very simple process or exercise. Put at its most concise, the essence of communication would appear to be the imparting, transmitting or sharing of some message or information between a sender and a receiver. Yet the reality of communication in nursing practice appears to be far from simple. Communication appears to cause many problems in nursing practice. Herein lies the paradox, for in theory, the act of communicating appears simple to understand and undertake, yet in reality it appears to cause nurses many difficulties (Argyle, 1981).

In order to understand the role of communication in a staff nurse's work, consider some of the roles a staff nurse will have to undertake during her everyday work. This list is not intended to be exhaustive, but is meant to demonstrate the importance of communication in the role of the staff nurse.

2.3. Communication and the role of the staff nurse

'The nursing care of the patient today makes great demands on nurses' knowledge and skills, especially if the care given is to be competent, efficient and effective.'

Bowman, M. (1986) p. 56

2.3.1. The staff nurse as clinician

A large part of any staff nurse's work involves the application of her clinical knowledge. In this role the staff nurse will be directly involved in the assessment, planning, implementation and evaluation of patient care. She will also be indirectly involved by way of supervising other nurses and in relaying information regarding, for example, a patient's condition, to medical or para-medical staff. In this area of her work, the staff nurse's ability to not only use (i.e., make decisions based on) her clinical knowledge, but also to communicate this knowledge in a clear concise manner to a number of potentially very different people is of obvious importance.

For example, when supervising or working with nurse learners the staff nurse will be attempting to impart or communicate her knowledge to the learner as clearly as possible, and in a manner most suited to the student's level of ability. In explaining procedures to patients or their relatives the staff nurse will attempt to communicate, in the most precise way possible, what is often very complex information. If the patient or his relative is left swimming in a sea of jargon or verbiage the nurse will have failed in her very important reassuring role. If clinical information is not communicated or only partially or inaccurately communicated, for example, between a nurse or doctor, or vice versa, then the results can be dangerous and on occasions fatal.

2.3.2. The staff nurse as ward organizer

The overall management and organization of a ward is important if it is to function properly. This can often appear rather mundane or repetitive work but it is nonetheless important ('petty management' as Florence Nightingale termed it). This involves the communication of diverse information from and to many diverse sources. The staff nurse has to liaise not only with the nurses working in the ward, but also with a wide range of other individuals and departments. In this role the staff nurse occupies an important focal position in ward organization. Much of the information which needs to be communicated in terms of the smooth running of the ward will be communicated through the staff nurse.

2.3.3. The staff nurse as personnel manager

Good management is as important as good organization for the effective functioning of a hospital ward, and good communication is an essential pre-requisite for good management. Good management implies that nurses are managed in a sensitive and mature manner, in an atmosphere which fosters high morale and values good patient care. This may be an ideal, but it is an ideal which is in the best interests of all those concerned.

In supervising, delegating, or planning the work of her staff, the staff nurse must attempt to ensure that first, she is being understood by those that she is managing and second, that she in turn understands and is sensitive to those she is managing. For good management to be practised the staff nurse must be a good communicator. Many nurses appear to blame low staffing levels or a bad environment for low morale. While these factors will undoubtedly have some bearing on morale, it appears that a common reason for failures in management at ward level is ineffective communication (Fretwell, 1982).

Failures in management may occur for a large number of reasons; for example, personality clashes, or a lack of a clearly defined line of responsibility. And yet, it is interesting to note that after two years experience of discussion and tutorials with staff nurses, the reason I have heard most frequently offered to explain what is perceived as poor management, is poor communication within the ward.

2.3.4. The staff nurse as information giver and receiver

Although aspects of this role are similar to that of the staff nurse as organizer it is worth investigating further to demonstrate the importance of communication in the transfer of information. The staff nurse will deal with large amounts of information, both verbal and written and, as previously mentioned, communicate this information to a wide variety of people or departments. The success, or otherwise, of the staff nurse in this role will depend to a large degree on her ability in three fields.

1. To collect information accurately.
2. To store it securely.
3. To ensure that the relevant information is passed on efficiently and precisely to the relevant person or department.

Many nurses may have experienced the problems which occur when information is not effectively communicated. For example, the patient arriving on the wrong day for his appointment. No matter what the precise cause of the communication failure may be, its effects can be dramatic. Again, the act of communicating can appear theoretically very simple, yet given the amount of verbal and written information which has to be given and received by the staff nurse, and the numbers of different people or groups to whom this must be passed on, the act of communicating, can, from a staff nurse's vantage point, appear most complex.

2.3.5. The staff nurse as 'Counsellor'

An important part of a staff nurse's work will be talking and listening to, or advising a large number of people: patients, their relatives, learner nurses, ancillary and domestic staff. Much of this work may be emotionally demanding: talking to a bereaved relative, chatting to a terminally ill patient, discussing a learner nurse's persistent lateness with her, or advising a young medical student about his bedside manner. Regardless of the form of counselling the staff nurse is undertaking, if it is to be effective the staff nurse must herself be an effective, thoughtful communicator.

This is not to suggest, however, that the use of the word counselling implies simply advising or disciplining someone. In its true meaning counselling implies a two-way therapeutic relationship. As Brearly and Birchley (1988) have commented on counselling skills, 'skills involved in enabling people to recognize their feelings, to define their problems and in helping people to find their own solutions or begin to resolve their dilemas are skills that can be developed by many people.'

Being aware of your own feelings and being sensitive enough to understand and empathize with the feelings and emotions of others is important, but not always easy. In addition to observing and actively listening to people, this process also involves encouraging other people to communicate. It may also involve questioning and responding appropriately or simply giving information. If the staff nurse is not receptive to other people's communications, or is unable to communicate effectively, then it may be that others will experience difficulty in communicating with her.

2.3.6. The staff nurse as 'Problem Solver'

If an emergency occurs in the ward when a staff nurse is in charge she will be expected to manage that emergency. She will be the person who will have to intervene and control any crisis which occurs when she is in charge. Overcoming or controlling any emergency requires good organization, and the staff nurse will have a crucial role to play in this situation. She will be responsible for assessing the situation, making decisions based on her assessment and then communicating those decisions to the relevant people or departments as soon as possible.

While dealing with an emergency the staff nurse will also have to maintain the smooth running of the ward, either by herself or by delegating to another. Thus the ability to communicate quickly and accurately, to take decisions and to assess, is of fundamental importance to the staff nurse's role in the management of an emergency.

2.3.7. The staff nurse as 'Assessor' and 'Decision-Maker'

It is not only as a problem-solver that the staff nurse will employ her skills of assessment and decision-making. She will be practising these whenever she is on duty. The staff nurse is required to make many decisions about many matters – she is required to make many judgements. For example, she may have to make a judgement or decision regarding a patient's physical condition, or a student nurse's fitness to continue nurse training. Whatever decision the nurse makes will be based upon the information she has available to her.

This information will be based on her own assessment of the situation, what she has observed herself, been told, or has gleaned from the written word. As a result her decisions can only be as thorough as the assessments upon which they are based. So that if the nurse is an effective communicator, both in terms of giving and receiving information, her performance as an assessor and decision-maker should be enhanced. If the nurse fails to receive and give information accurately, her abilities as a decision-maker may well suffer.

2.3.8. The staff nurse as the 'Patient's Advocate'

Often, nurses in all areas of activity may nurse people who can do, or say, very little for themselves. In line with the UKCC Code of Conduct it is therefore a nurse's responsibility to act as an advocate, ('to defend or plead') (Concise OED) for a patient who cannot do so for himself. Here, it is important to be sensitive to a patient's potentially impaired communications. The nurse should attempt to understand the patient's needs so that she can then communicate these to other people more effectively. If nurses are to be able to speak on behalf of those in their care, they must be confident that they truly understand patients' needs and are conveying these accurately.

The foregoing discussion is not intended to suggest that a staff nurse's job can or should be artificially compartmentalized into its component roles. In reality the staff nurse may well be acting many or all of these roles simultaneously. Three factors emerge which are important in the further consideration of communication.

Firstly, the central role which the staff nurse plays in ward organization and management. Secondly, the sometimes stressful nature of her work. Much research has been carried out into the nature of stress in nursing. There appears to be considerable agreement that nursing can be a stressful occupation, see Bond (1986) and Menzies (1970) for example. Thirdly, it would appear that if a staff nurse is not an effective communicator, then virtually all other aspects of her work may suffer.

Bearing in mind these three factors we will now consider the subject of communication in greater depth.

2.4. What is effective communication?

'When we describe communication we are really discussing human relationships. When we interpret others' efforts to relate to us or when we analyse our own efforts to relate to others, we are communicating . . . To understand the process of communication we must understand how people relate to each other.'

Bass, A. (1982) p. 6

The essence of communication was defined earlier as the imparting, transmitting or sharing of some message or information between a sender and a receiver. Employing this definition in considering a staff nurse's work we find that effective communication for her means that she is able effectively to impart, transmit or share messages and information with other people or groups, herself being both a sender and receiver of information.

The better to understand what effective communication means in practice we will now explore some of the important aspects of communication. Given the very varied work of nurses, the uniqueness of each individual and the uniqueness of every situation in which communication occurs, it is only really possible to outline or suggest guidelines. It may be possible to state policy or rules for given situations, yet there is a danger of creating an automaton-like dullness, which stultifies naturalness and creativity in communications.

As with the review of the staff nurse's role these aspects are not intended to be exhaustive, but seek to outline the major factors involved in effective communication. Thoughtfully applied however, they should be universally applicable. They will be considered under four headings.

1. General aspects.
2. Aspects affecting verbal communication.
3. Aspects affecting non-verbal communication.
4. Aspects affecting written communication.

2.4.1. General aspects

Consistency

This will affect all areas of a staff nurse's behaviour and hence communications. The Concise Oxford Dictionary defines consistent as 'compatable, not contradictory, constant to same principles'. (Concise OED). This is not to suggest that a staff nurse should behave in a completely robot-like, rigid way, all the time. Her behaviour, like that of everyone else around her, may vary according to many psychological and physical factors. What is important, as the definition states, is that she should not contradict. It is normal to allow for changes in mood in other people, indeed we may gradually learn that some people's moods appear more volatile than others.

What is very upsetting is to approach somebody who is normally 'all sweetness and light' only to find that they respond with uncharacteristic anger. Many nurses may have experienced working with someone in a position of authority who appears to have marked changes of mood. If so, they will know the damage this can do to good communications. Younger or less experienced nurses may be unsure or nervous of the person in charge and everyone has to wait and see 'what she's going to be like today'. If, as a staff nurse, you are in charge, you should try to ensure that the people to whom you relate always feel free and able to communicate with you.

Observation

In order to carry out many aspects of her work the staff nurse must be able to observe accurately and thoughtfully all that is important around her. Obviously the nurse cannot be expected to know everything that is happening; rather she should know what factors to observe in the ward around her. The staff nurse should also make her observations as constant as possible, and attempt to think constructively about what she has seen.

The ability to observe intelligently is important in all three areas of communication. For example, in non-verbal communication, are you a good observer of people's facial expressions, their eye contact (or lack of it), their body language? In verbal communication – can you accurately evaluate somebody's speech, including accent, pitch, and speed? In written communication, do you observe case notes accurately, can you spot a faulty or dubious prescription in a drug kardex? Observation, then, is a most important part of effective communication. Not only will it aid assessment and decision-making, it should also aid the staff nurse in all aspects of her work.

Courtesy

This may, at first, appear a rather old-fashioned word, yet its meaning is very relevant to the communication skills of a staff nurse, namely, 'polite, kind, considerate in manner and address' (Concise OED). As suggested the staff nurse can occupy a focal position in ward communication. She may have to communicate with many different people and may be a role model for learner nurses.

For example, a staff nurse who verbally 'snaps' at a patient, when a considered gentle answer would have been more appropriate, may have had a number of reasons for doing so. She may have been tired, or harassed, or found that particular patient difficult to deal with. However, even though many (or all) of these reasons may be valid, they do not excuse her momentary lapse. It may indeed be extremely difficult to remain courteous in some situations, when under stress or provocation for example. But it appears that, like it or not, the staff nurse must set an example. This is especially so in using yourself as a role model for good communications.

That nurses need at least to attempt to be courteous is well documented. As Darbyshire (1988) states when discussing nurses' dissatisfaction with their job: 'If there is one feature which seems to underpin these expressions of dissatisfaction, it is the feeling many nurses share that they are treated with considerably less than due respect in their place of work.' He continues, 'It is probably significant that the reasons given by most nurses for leaving relate to the poor quality of relationships at their place of work.' Courtesy of itself will not solve the problems of interpersonal relationships, but bearing in mind the principle of courtesy should positively aid relationships and hence communication.

Organization

Just as good communication is important to good organization, so good organization is a pre-requisite for effective communication. In any type of ward there will be a constant flow of verbal and written information moving in and out of the ward, and much of this may pass through the nurse in charge. If the person in charge happens to be a staff nurse, then she will be responsible for the smooth transmission of this information.

A major element in this process will be the organization of information. For effective communication to occur, things must be organized so as to encourage communication, rather than hinder it. If information does not appear to be moving around smoothly, then it may be that some organizational change is necessary, to encourage a more efficient flow of information. If you yourself are well organized, then not only will your abilities as a communictor be improved but the whole of your nursing practice should benefit.

Confidence

A staff nurse's own level of confidence may have a tremendous effect on her ability to communicate with others, and their ability to communicate with her. A loud bombastic staff nurse may appear over-confident to some patients, who may therefore be discouraged from communicating with her. Likewise patients may not communicate with a staff nurse whom they perceive as so weak and lacking in confidence that she cannot get anything done for them. Obviously, both extremes are to be avoided.

Yet people normally find confidence through experience, they gain it through learning. Even though the new staff nurse may not, in reality feel very confident in her new and alien role, she must at least attempt to appear confident for the sake of those around her. This is in no way to suggest that she should adopt a false exterior confidence, or take risks with patients in the name of confidence, without really knowing what she is doing. However, if the person in charge of the ward is perceived by patients or colleagues to be lacking in confidence, or unsure of her judgements, this may have a serious effect on communications within the ward.

While the new staff nurse will hopefully gain confidence as she gains experience in her new role, she should at least have the confidence of knowing where and how she can gain assistance or support if required. For as the staff nurse gains confidence, in her own knowledge, in managing staff, in relating to medical staff, or in dealing with relatives, so her ability to communicate effectively should improve.

Sensitivity

In discussing the roles of the staff nurse it was suggested that sensitivity was often required to do her job effectively. It is also a principle of effective communication. Sensitivity is defined as 'readily responding to, or, recording slight changes of condition' (Concise OED). The staff nurse should therefore know what factors are important, i.e., what factors should be watched for and hence responded to. The staff nurse should also be aware or sensitive enough to notice or observe any slight changes in a person's condition, mood or behaviour.

For example, if a staff nurse is giving a verbal report on a patient's condition this report will be more meaningful if the nurse has spent time with the patient, observing all aspects of his person as keenly as possible. Spending time with patients and observing them will not of itself help nurses to be more sensitive to the mood, behaviour or physical condition of other people. What is important is that when with a patient, a nurse should observe him as accurately as possible, and react as sensitively as possible to what the patient is communicating to her.

The nurse should be able to note the many small features of behaviour which may indicate that a patient is in some way unhappy or upset. For example quickened speech, jumpy eye-contact or a rigid physical position. Given that hospitals may be highly stressful places, it is vital that staff nurses be able both to observe people in a sensitive manner and to react sensitively to their physical and emotional needs.

Humour

Regardless of the mode of communication, humour, if employed thoughtfully and tactfully, may greatly enhance communication. Equally, if used tactlessly, humour may turn a difficult situation into a nightmare. A light-hearted remark from a staff nurse to a patient in one situation may have great positive value in relieving that patient's anxiety. However, the same aside in a different situation may serve only to heighten a patient's anxiety, a situation not conducive to effective communication.

Although the term, 'a sense of humour', may simply imply the telling or appreciation of jokes, it is used here in a broader sense. In this sense it implies a general cheerfulness or geniality on the part of the nurse. If a staff nurse is known by those in her care to possess these qualities, it is more likely that effective communication will occur. Similarly, if a staff nurse is seen as being cold or humourless, this may hinder her effectiveness as a communicator. There are obviously times in nursing when seriousness is perfectly in order, yet on many other occasions even a smile from a nurse can greatly aid her role as communicator.

2.4.2. Aspects relevant to verbal communication

Clarity and precision

Much of a staff nurse's day may be taken up in giving and receiving verbal communications. Due to her role in the ward the staff nurse will be required to communicate verbally a large amount of often complex verbal information, with many different people. It is therefore important that the staff nurse attempts to ensure that those around her really understand what she is communicating to them.

The staff nurse's chances of being understood by those around her will be much enhanced if she can make her communications as clear and precise as possible. However, there may be impediments to good verbal communications over which the staff nurse has no control, for example, a patient's hearing difficulty, or a very noisy telephone line. Yet the staff nurse can go a long way to overcoming these problems by firstly considering exactly whom it is she is talking to, and secondly keeping her communications as clear and precise as possible.

Attentive listening

This may appear to be a rather mundane factor to discuss as a principle, but is a vitally important part of effective verbal communication. Just as it is important to observe people physically, so it is important to observe them aurally. In getting to know someone with whom she works, the staff nurse may learn a lot

from good physical observation, yet she may learn a ⎰
more about the person simply by listening to him.

The ability to listen to others is important in a number ⎰
It should aid assessment, for the more knowledge a nurse can
gain about someone, the more thorough should be the assessment.
It should also aid a nurse's conversation skills, for if she can
patiently let people 'have their say' and respond sensitively, more
effective communication should ensue. To be truly effective, listening should be undertaken in an active manner. The nurse should
try to take time and effort to demonstrate that she is really paying
attention to what is being said to her. If someone with whom the
nurse is involved, gets the impression that the nurse is talking to
her merely 'in passing', the quality of communication may well
suffer.

2.4.3. Aspects relevant to 'non-verbal communication'
Many writers on this subject of communication, Argyle, for example, have suggested (1979) that there is a larger non-verbal than
verbal component to communication. In short we communicate
more through our bodies, faces, or eyes than through our mouths.
This is clearly an important part of a nurse's communication skills.

Awareness of 'facial expressions'
There are more independent muscle groups in the face than in
any other part of the body. This is clearly visible in the large
number of facial expressions which can be observed when people
are communicating. In fact, the face alone can convey a large
number of emotions – anger, mirth, resignation, determination –
to name but four. It will therefore help the staff nurse greatly, in
her attempts to understand someone else's communications if she
is aware of and sensitive to people's facial expressions.

Awareness of 'bodily position'
Just as the nurse may learn about someone's mood by observing
his facial expression, so she may gain a greater understanding by
observing his whole body. Our body's position or stance may
often reflect our inner emotions. For example, standing in a very
rigid manner wringing hands may imply nervousness, or sitting
on the ground in a slouched position, with head between the
knees may imply extreme fatigue. With a keen awareness and
understanding of bodily communication, often termed body lan-

guage, the staff nurse will be better equipped to understand what patients may be communicating to her.

Awareness of 'eye-contact'

Although romantically referred to as 'windows of the soul', the eyes, are very important in communication. As with the face and body, many emotions may be expressed through the eyes. Eye-contact is also very important in conversation. Between sighted people, eye-contact is a pre-requisite for conversation, and indeed we continue to use our eyes to communicate throughout the conversation. People may cast their eyes downwards in shame, or raise their eyes quickly heavenwards to indicate some form of frustration. On some occasions eye contact may be a positive form of communication in its own right. For example a warm and supportive glance from a nurse may help to communicate reassurance to a worried patient.

2.4.4. Aspects relevant to written communication

Written communication is an important part of the communication process. Although it may sound rather Victorian, when applied sensibly, the principles of good writing can greatly aid communication.

Neatness, legibility and clarity

These terms may sound more like the exhortations of a primary school teacher to her class, but they are none the less vital to effective written communication. If a staff nurse's hand-writing and general paperwork is consistently ordered, understandable and readable, then there will be far less chance of others misunderstanding her written communication.

The need for accurate written communication is particularly important in the areas of drug administration and recording nursing care. One only needs to refer to the proceedings of the UKCC Disciplinary Committee to see the sometimes tragic results of failures in this area of communication. Even though she possesses excellent verbal and non-verbal communication abilities, her skills as a communicator will be greatly impaired if she cannot communicate equally well through the written word.

Self-awareness

'Nursing is stressful work, and while some stress is stimulating, too much can make you feel sick and unhappy. Stress is a problem for nurses as they tend to put other people's problems before their own.'

Bond, M. (1986)

There would appear to be two means by which the staff nurse may improve her abilities as a communicator. The first is to make good any deficiencies she may have regarding her knowledge of communication. As a nurse's knowledge of a subject grows, so should her understanding and awareness of that subject. The second is simply to get to know herself better, for it appears that communication can be improved by increased self-awareness. Burnard (1985) describes this idea saying, 'nurses must deal with other people's emotions, and there is a positive link between the way in which we handle our own emotions and the way in which we handle those of others. If we understand and appropriately express our own anger, grief, fear and embarrassment, we will be better able to handle them in other people. In caring for others we must get to know ourselves better.'

What is self-awareness?

Self-awareness is not easily defined. It is not a quality which one person may possess and another may not. We will all be aware of ourselves to some degree or other. The important point regarding the concept of self-awareness is the degree to which we are aware of ourselves. Consider this definition: 'Self-awareness refers to the gradual and continuous process of noticing and explaining aspects of self whether behavioural, psychological or personal and interpersonal understanding' (Burnard, 1985). It will be noted here that self-awareness requires that we look inwards on ourselves, not in an indulgent 'navel-gazing' manner, but with the purpose of improving our outward understanding and so hopefully our communication abilities.

Given the uniqueness of every individual it would be very difficult, in any hard and fast way, to state what self-awareness would mean to each individual. What can be stated though, is the possible benefits for all individuals which may accrue through increased self-awareness. Through greater self-awareness the nurse should be better able to differentiate between her own feelings and those of others. If she is unable to, then she may be 'swallowed-up' in a patient's anguish or fear, and be of little real help to him. Equally, if a nurse is battling to cope with her own emotions, she may be unable to give of her best to those in her care, and so communications may well suffer. Increased self-awareness should lead to greater tolerance on the part of the nurse. If we are aware of and at peace with both our strengths and weaknesses, then we should be more understanding of the 'pluses and minuses' in others.

If the nurse is well aware of her own professional strengths and weaknesses, then hopefully she may be more understanding of the same factors in her colleagues. In this way she may become more sensitive to giving support and guidance when required, actions which may greatly aid effective communication. Self-awareness is also very important in terms of image; for whatever image a nurse presents will have a great effect on her communications.

For example the nurse who is perceived as being friendly and approachable should be able to communicate more effectively than the nurse who is perceived as being cold or unapproachable. It is, therefore, in the interests of the nurse to be well aware of her own image. With a greater awareness of how she is perceived, she should be able to communicate more effectively. And with a good awareness of her own feelings the nurse should be in a position to empathize with patients and colleagues, an ability which can greatly aid communication.

Whatever one's route to increased self-awareness may be, the process has to begin at a personal level. We should start by asking ourselves many questions, for we must be able to look at ourselves in the mirror, 'warts and all'. We must try to develop an increased awareness of, for example, our personality, our experience, our image, our attitudes (are we aware of any negative attitudes we possess which may interfere with our relationships and hence communications with patients and colleagues?) and we should attempt to identify our own strengths and weaknesses and, more importantly, come to terms with them. This process will be point-less if undertaken in a spirit of self-indulgence. Rather, it should be undertaken with the understanding that greater self-awareness should lead to an improved ability to relate to and hence communi-cate with others.

Discussing the development of self-awareness Burnard (1985) highlights three important points. Firstly, the voluntariness of self-awareness. For the process to be meaningful each individual should have the freedom to develop awareness at her own pace; 'self-awareness cannot be forced on people.' Secondly, the problem of egocentricity. As stated the purpose of this exercise is to enable us to relate better to those around us, not simply selfishly looking in upon ourselves. Thirdly, the danger of possibly becoming over serious or pompous as a result of our new-found awareness. As Burnard puts it, ' . . . those who adopt the (false) sense of the wise person can be notoriously humourless and earnest. True self-awareness more usually brings a sense of humility and awe at the sheer vastness of the task undertaken.'

There may be a number of potential routes to increased self-awareness. For example, discussion groups between staff, awareness courses, or 'brain-storming' sessions. Simple observation is another possible route to increased self-awareness, for if we can observe others' behaviour, and how they cope in difficult situations, it may be possible – with reflection – to learn more about ourselves. Open discussion with colleagues and peers may be another route to increased self-awareness, for if nurses can share their own worries, doubts or uncertainties, a greater understanding of others and ourselves may result.

In conclusion, communication is a large and important subject which is crucial to all aspects of a staff nurse's role. A failure in a nurse's communications may well adversely affect all other aspects of her work. However, with a healthy self-awareness and a confident grasp of the principles of communication, the staff nurse should be better placed to be a competent practitioner and adept communicator.

References

Argyle, M. (1981) *Social Skills and Health*, Methuen, London.

Argyle, M. (1975) *Bodily Communication*, Methuen, London.

Argyle, M. and Trower, P. (1979) *Person to Person*, Harper and Row, London.

Bass, A. and Smith, V. (1982) in *Communication for the Health Care Team* (ed. A. Faulkner), Harper and Row, London.

Blonds, M. and Jackson, B. (1982) *Non-verbal Communications with Patients*, John Wiley and Sons, New York.

Bond, M. (1986) *Stress and Self Awareness: A Guide for Nurses*, Heinemann, London.

Bowman, M. (1986) *Nursing Management and Education*, Croom Helm, London.

Brearley, G. and Birchley, G. (1988) *Introducing Counselling Skills and Techniques*, Faber and Faber, London.

Burton, G. (1979) *Interpersonal Relations*, Tavistock, London.

Burnard, P. (1985) *Learning Human Skills*, Heinemann, London.

Darbyshire, P. (1988) Thinly Disguised Contempt, *Nursing Times*, **84** (20) pp 42–44.

Faulkner, A. (1984) *Communication*, Churchill Livingstone, Edinburgh.

Fretwell, J. (1982) *Ward Teaching and Learning*, RCN, London.

Hargie, O. Saunders, C. and Dickson, D. (1981) *Social Skills in Interpersonal Communication*, Croom Helm, London.

Kagan, C. Evans, J. and Kay, B. (1986) *Interpersonal Skills for Nurses*, Harper and Row, London.

Kagan, C. (Ed.) (1985) *Interpersonal Skills in Nursing*, Croom Helm, London.

Menzies, M. (1970) *Defence Systems as a Control Against Anxiety*, Tavistock, London.

Pope, B. (1986) *Social Skills Training for Psychiatric Nurses*, Harper and Row, London.

Rogers, W. (1984) *Communication in Action*, Holt, Rinehart and Winston, New York.

3

Working in and with groups

Dirjodhun Mojee

3.1. Introduction

An awareness and understanding of group behaviour, as distinct from individual behaviour, is important to the staff nurse in her role as manager and teacher. It helps to identify positive group behaviours, and to highlight problems that the group may be experiencing. Identification of such behaviours, and having the skill to lead the nursing team successfully, benefits both the staff nurse, and as a result the patient.

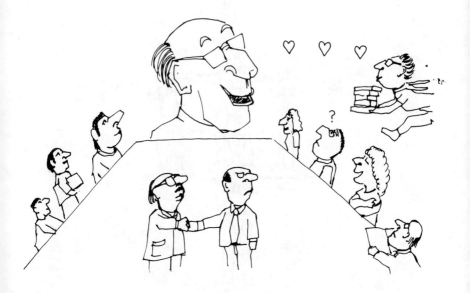

Figure 3.1 Group behaviour – positive or negative!

Identification of positive and negative behaviours may not be an easy task, as each group as an entity differs in some ways from other groups. However, there are certain behaviours that are found in all groups. Conflicts and support between members are present in a nursing group as much as a brick-laying squad. It is hoped that by understanding these positive and negative behaviours the staff nurse's ability to lead and participate in groups will be enhanced.

We spend much of our working or social life in one group setting or another. A staff nurse may spend up to about 50% of her working time either leading or participating in a group. Such groups may be ward meetings, multi-disciplinary meetings, teaching and learning groups and patient support groups. In recent years organizations are recognizing that good teamwork is essential for two reasons.

1. To improve the quality of life, in the case of nursing, care for the patient.

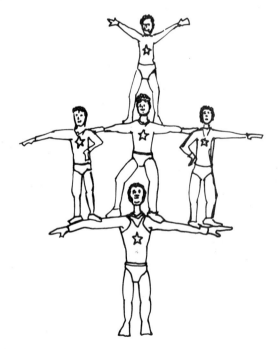

Figure 3.2   A group

2. To improve job satisfaction, and therefore morale, in staff of all ranks.

The intention in this chapter is to shed some light on what groups are, why they are needed and how they operate. It is hoped that by generating this awareness, the staff nurse will be better placed to lead a team.

3.2. What is a group?

By definition, a group is a collection of three or more people who meet and interact on a regular basis for a purpose.

Groups can be informal, when a loose collection of friends meet on an irregular basis at work or in a public house. Groups can also be formal, when there is a set number of people who meet on a regular basis, such as tutorial groups, ward staff meetings, multi-disciplinary groups. In such groups there are usually set or implied objectives, and in most cases an outcome is expected. By implication, therefore, a loose collection of people who wait at a bus stop is not either a formal or informal group; it is a non-group.

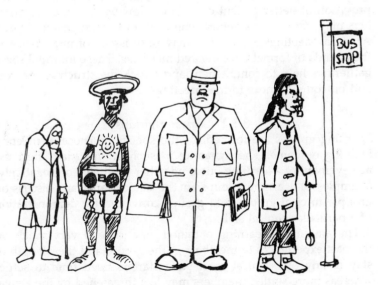

Figure 3.3 A non-group

3.3. Group types

There are broadly two types of groups in health care.

1. Work groups.
2. Learning groups.

3.3.1. Work groups

As part of their normal span of duty, nursing staff may be called upon to participate in one or more work groups. These may take the form of committees, working groups or case conferences. In times of change there tends to be a proliferation of working groups. For example, at the moment there are various working groups in hospitals and colleges of nursing looking at Quality Assurance and the transition in nursing education to Project 2000. The common thread among all these groups is that they are established for specific purposes, with specific remits.

Individuals in the workplace do meet informally for various reasons which may not be directly work-related. These informal meetings help to improve relationships in such groups, and therefore directly enrich the character of formal work-related groups. For example, the specific purpose of ward meetings may be the provision of better patient care, but following the meeting members may stay on for a general chit-chat, or to arrange a night out. At social meetings individuals may raise issues of importance to the agenda of formal work-related meetings. These informal social gatherings help to complement and enrich the structure, process and outcome of more formal meetings.

3.3.2. Learning groups

Learning groups are formed for the specific purpose of meeting learning outcome. The dynamics in such groups may affect the achievement of a learning outcome either positively or negatively. Examples of learning groups in the clinical area are discussion groups, tutorial groups and groups convened for demonstration of a particular clinical skill.

The amount of learning obtained may depend very much on the past experiences of members in the group, and their length of stay in any one clinical area. New starters need time to settle, whereas more settled members may feel threatened by the arrival of new members who may get equal or more support from trained

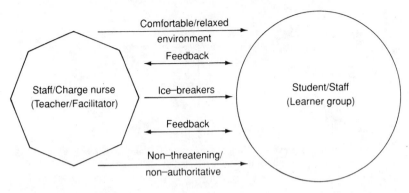

Figure 3.4 The teacher/learning interraction

members of staff. Until their anxieties are rationalized the learning outcome may be affected. It is helpful if the ward has a clearly defined programme of induction that students or newly trained staff have to go through. This helps to relieve anxieties because everyone is aware that extra support to new members is not synonymous with less support for others, but part of normal ward policy.

Trained staff who are involved in clinical teaching need to be aware that, where groups are concerned, time must be allowed for the group members to know each other before they get down to the actual task of teaching or learning. This may be done in several ways, including the following.

1. Use of ice-breakers.
2. Creating a comfortable and relaxed environment.
3. Projecting a non-threatening, non-authoritative attitude.

3.4. Need for knowledge in group dynamics

Working in and with groups is a way of life for most managers, those in health care being no exception. Managers spend a considerable amount of time either leading or participating in one group or another. These groups may take the form of formal unit or ward meetings, or multi-disciplinary meetings where patient's progress may be discussed. When such groups meet, the potential for contribution from both individuals and the group are considerable, given that the right atmosphere and environment prevails.

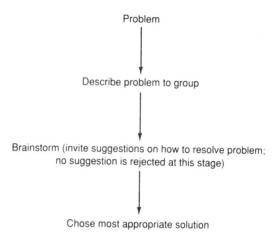

Problem

Describe problem to group

Brainstorm (invite suggestions on how to resolve problem;
no suggestion is rejected at this stage)

Chose most appropriate solution

Figure 3.5 The brainstorming process

Each member in such groups brings experiences which may be of immense use to the group. 'Tapping' for ideas makes use of such experiences. 'Brainstorming' is one way commonly used to 'tap' for ideas.

Problems are described to group members. Ideas about solutions to the problems are invited. No suggestion is rejected, however irrational. Once the 'brainstormed' ideas have been collected, then the group helps in deciding which solution is the most appropriate. Brainstorming for ideas may be worth a try in the clinical setting. You may be amazed at the variety of suggestions you may get from your staff.

A group may be a rich source of ideas, but to get the best out of group members the leader needs a knowledge of group dynamics, and the skill to manage the group to best effect. Some skills of primary benefit are sound social and interpersonal skills. So, what is group dynamics? Group dynamics consists of behaviours demonstrated by the group during meetings and normal deliberations. Examples are collective support or rejection of the appointed leader, or sub-group formation, ('cliques'). Then there are the 'passive' ones, the 'know-it-alls', and the 'chronic complainers'. One positive dynamic that most groups display is collective responsibility and 'power'. Because individuals feel that any decision made is the responsibility of the group, they feel less

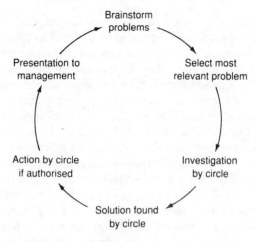

Figure 3.6 How the quality circle operates

inhibited to participate. Collective responsibility gives the group 'power'.

The ability to generate new ideas, and the collective responsibility and power that groups display, can be put to good use by ward managers. 'Quality Circles', which are ward-based groups formed to find solutions to work-based problems, provide a good example of the potential that groups have, and the commitment they can show if they are consulted and their suggestions are valued.

Quality circles are 'a structured way of making management listen'. The phrase used in Japan is 'a gathering of the wisdom of the people'! It involves not more than twelve members meeting fortnightly to solve work-related problems. It uses a 'bottom-up' approach, in so far as the worker identifies the problem, and finds a solution to it. The solution is then presented for management to act upon. The circle starts with a 'moaning session'. Problems are identified and prioritized. Constructive and sensible solutions are then put forward. The benefit of this approach is that when people are involved from the very outset in decisions about their own work, this increases their commitment. Increased commitment may lead to an improvement in the quality of the service offered. This may then lead to job satisfaction and an uplifting of morale.

Exchange of ideas, new ways of doing things, how different

members have dealt with different problems, the success and failure of past practices and processes, all tend to produce a fertile ground for learning. Learning groups are not different from work groups in certain aspects. They display similar dynamics, and they both undergo a process of maturation. Individuals' aspirations for the future are shared. Members get the opportunity to compare expectations and aspirations. Knowles (1970) observed this process and coined the term 'Participatory Learning'. He describes it thus: 'The adult learner is more self-directing, is a reservoir of experience and resource. The adult learner is orientated towards problem-centered learning rather than subject-centered; that is "the theoretical" must have a "practical outlet". The "practical outlet" is richer because of the reservoir of experiences that individuals bring to groups. The responsibility of the group leader, who may be a teacher or a trained nurse in the clinical situation, is to ease the flow of these experiences through discussion and general socialization.'

There is a social outcome to belonging to any group. Although some members may avoid such socialization, most positively seek and seal friendships to the mutual enjoyment of the parties concerned. Festinger (1963), proposed a 'theory of social comparison'. The theory proposes that people want to, and need to compare their opinions, abilities and potentials with others. There seems to exist a subtle, healthy 'competition' among group members. Individuals observe each other, and try to either emulate or outdo each other. This 'peer group pressure' pushes members towards conformity. Those members who find it difficult to conform, either try to change the 'rules', or leave.

The reasons, therefore, for group leaders, teachers, supervisors to have a thorough knowledge of group processes are many. Such knowledge helps in understanding the variety of behaviours, both negative and positive that groups display. The leader may then be better equipped to use the appropriate skills to get the most out of groups they are leading.

3.5. Tuckman's model of group life

When groups meet for the first time, they go through a process of development and maturity. However diverse the composition of the group in terms of age, experience and background, it still progresses through set stages of development. Tuckman (1973) observed this phenomenon and developed a model to explain it. The model divides the maturing process into five stages. The five stages cover the period from the time the group convenes to the time they disband, or they are settled enough to start working on the task in hand.

1. Forming stage – Own code of conduct.
2. Storming stage – It can't be done / I won't do it.
3. Norming stage – We can do it.
4. Performing stage – We are doing it.
5. Ending stage – Leave group / May meet again.

3.5.1. Forming stage

The group is a collection of people with very little in common. There is exchange of names, likes and dislikes. Members tend to be hesitant, and are more involved in observing each other, although very discreetly. However, because of the physical closeness and presence of members, conversation is initiated. The initiative to converse may be taken by one of the more extrovert members, or an introvert one where it may be anxiety-led. The more passive members tend to react to the 'social chit-chat'. Disclosure of feelings and opinions is very low because of lack of trust. This warming-up stage is an important process in Tuckman's model of group life. Teachers and group leaders are well aware of this stage, because minimal learning or work takes place at this stage. The teacher should attempt to use 'ice-breakers' to facilitate a group of students through this stage. The learning environment should be such that the group feels relaxed and convivial. The

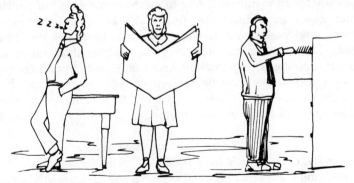

Figure 3.7   Group life – Forming stage

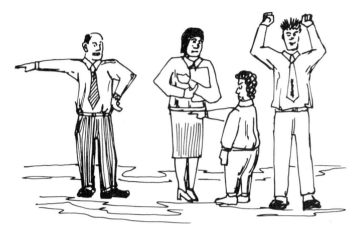

Figure 3.8   Group life – Storming stage

group leader or supervisor may find that the 'productive capacity' of the group is limited at this stage. It is therefore essential for group leaders and teachers to help their groups through this stage before they start on the task in hand, be it educational or work-related.

3.5.2. Storming stage

This stage may be a traumatic one for the group. It brings out the differences rather than the similarities in the group. Members in the group explore what is unique or different about other members. There may be verbal and non-verbal friction and 'infighting', associated with members trying to establish some sort of pecking order. Some individuals may find that their aspirations, expectations, and needs conflict with other members' and the group needs. Each member may join the group with an individual 'package' of aspirations, expectations and needs, only to find that the group's aspirations may be in conflict with theirs. Until these aspirations and needs are congruent, there may be minimal achievement in terms of task or learning.

3.5.3. Norming stage

By this stage individuals have tried, and in most cases succeeded, in resolving the conflict between personal and group needs. Group needs may now be perceived as more valuable than individual

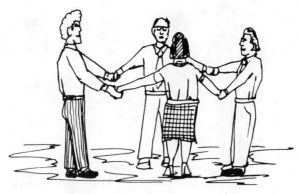

Figure 3.9 Group life – Norming stage

personal needs. If they are not, then individuals may carry those forward as 'hidden agendas', and bring them up from time to time during deliberations. The group starts to 'set'. It starts to develop a character of its own. The group character may reflect the sum total of the individual members' characters in the group. No two ward teams or student groups show the same aspirations, enthusiasm or subculture. No two groups are alike. This fact is of importance to teachers and group leaders. The group may at this stage establish its own 'rules', its *modus operandi*. There may be more cohesion, in terms of there being more agreements on issues than disagreements. Individuals start identifying themselves as being part of the group; and therefore, may be prepared to defend the group's policies and agenda when and if these are challenged by people outside the group.

3.5.4. Performing stage

By this stage the group has 'come of age'. Differences will have been resolved or perceived as less important than group unity. The group has reached its productive stage. More time and effort is spent dealing with the task in hand. If there are any lingering individual differences or conflict of purpose, these tend to be accepted by group members as insignificant. Group leaders and teachers need to be aware of the importance of this stage in group development. Until this stage is reached, it may not be possible to gain the interest and enthusiasm of the group. The group will need to be helped through the earlier stages before the task in hand is tackled. The time, effort and patience spent in facilitation

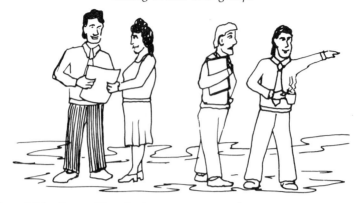

Figure 3.10 Group life – Performing stage

is worthwhile. This may take the form of full introduction of group members to each other; every member being clear about the objectives of the group; each member being seen as important and valuable potential contributors to the group's objectives. A comfortable and relaxed environment may help the process.

3.5.5. Ending stage

At this stage the group disbands, unless it is a group of students on a lengthy course, or members of a working group with an ongoing remit in a college of nursing or hospital. As members leave, they leave behind both pleasant and unpleasant memories of their experiences in the group. By and large, however, friendships develop, and individuals may see each other again for social reasons.

It is important to recognize that groups differ from each other because of their composition, location, length of time they are together, and the leadership style of the teacher or leader who leads the group. Different groups may take different amounts of time proceeding through the different stages. Length of time spent in each stage also depends on whether or not members joined the group by choice or compulsion. The skilled teacher or group leader can help in 'easing' the group through the different stages, thereby reducing the time taken to reach the performing stage.

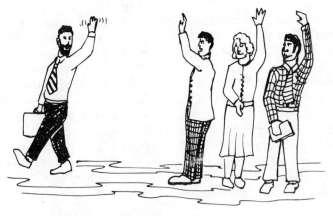

Figure 3.11 Group life – Ending stage

3.6. Possible behaviours in groups

Groups, being diverse in character, present many possibilities in terms of behaviours projected. The type and composition of the group can affect the behaviour outcome of each individual. An individual participating in a multi-disciplinary meeting may behave differently from when in a group with people of similar grade on a leadership course. Behaviours tend to be specific to a situation at a specific time. The same individual, put in a similar situation at a different time may behave differently. The range of behaviours, therefore, can be varied and unexpected. Hence, whoever is leading a group needs to have knowledge of group dynamics, and the skill to facilitate the group in the desired direction.

Individual members bring to the group their own needs and expectations. As the group settles, these needs and expectations blend and emerge as the group needs and expectations. Each new member who joins the group puts the group through a mini crisis, when adjustment and accommodation may take place. When the group is in a settled state, it holds a certain set of behaviours as 'normal'. The group has certain norms, a set of expected modes of behaviour and beliefs that are specific to the group. There may be sanctions for infringement of group norms. These norms may cover such aspects of nursing activities as standard of patient care, good or bad housekeeping or annual leave arrangements for staff.

For example, an individual whose standard is low may be pressurized to 'toe the line' on joining a group where standard of patient care is high. Acceptance within a group demands conformity.

Awareness of group norms and adherence to them, gives cohesion to a group. In theory, cohesion should be to the benefit of the group. Individuals feel settled and valued. This may improve performance in terms of quality and quantity of work produced. However, too much cohesion can be counterproductive. It reduces the likelihood of exploring different ways of doing things or solving problems. There may be cohesion at the expense of quality, if low standard work is the norm for the group. Healthy confrontation, therefore, may be the balance to aim for in terms of group dynamics.

Confrontation can be of value to the group. Catastrophic and undesirable decisions may be the result of lack of confrontation. Although cohesion may lead to a decrease in absenteeism and more job satisfaction, members may avoid raising controversial and contentious issues, or questioning weak arguments. Too much confrontation, however, can lead to the group breaking up; whereas too much cohesion can lead to insufficient exploration of ideas or courses of action.

Another dynamic in a group's life is the formation of hierarchies. Individuals may set, or move up or down within that hierarchy. Movement tends to depend on a member's age, job characteristic, social presence and sex. Ward teams, for example, may exemplify a hierarchy in the following way. The charge nurse, being the formal leader, may be at the top of the pecking order because of job status, age and length of service. Next in the hierarchy may be the staff nurses. However, if there is a power vacuum because of weak leadership, a staff nurse may be perceived as the leader by the rest of the group because of her superior expertise and social presence. If the charge nurse is not seen to manage the task of patient care well, the staff may direct part of their allegiance to lower-ranked members in the group. These may be staff nurses or enrolled nurses.

Leadership, therefore is vital to a group in terms of its dynamics. Leadership, or the lack of it, affects the group's efficiency, productivity and satisfaction. The style of leadership used in a particular situation may be autocratic, democratic or *laissez-faire*.

The best style is the one most appropriate to the situation or the group. An interesting study by White and Lippitt (1960) observed the result of using different leadership styles. Youngsters were exposed to classes led by teachers using each of the above three styles. The autocratic teacher 'told' the class what to do. The children in this instance spent more time working, but the work rate dropped off as soon as the teacher left the room. Some of the children from this group later destroyed the work they had so painstakingly produced. Those children who were exposed to the *laissez-faire* styled teacher, who told them they could do whatever they pleased, spent most of the time playing around or simply loafing. However, those children who were led by the democratic teacher, where they had some say in what they were to do, kept working even when the teacher was not there. They also produced better work than both the other groups, and they showed more interest in their activity. Although this study used children to show the three styles in action, it does exemplify the outcome of using different styles of leadership.

Children's behaviour, however, tends to be spontaneous. When considering adult groups, where behaviour is more controlled and purposeful, the appropriate style to use would depend on the group and the type of situation it is in. In times of crisis, such as an outbreak of fire or a cardiac arrest, whoever leads the situation can only be autocratic in approach. However, where time is not short, and safety of patient or staff is not an issue, there is no reason why a leader should not adopt a *laissez-faire* approach, especially when dealing with a mature and trusted group, where each individual is clear about group goals and objectives.

In developmental terms, groups are dynamic. Leadership is interactive. The leadership style used by the leader depends on the task in hand, the maturity of the group, and the situation the group is in. Leadership, therefore, matters in group dynamics. Styles of leadership affect the quality and the quantity of the work produced, the satisfaction people get out of belonging to a group and the continuity and stability of the group in the absence of the leader. The staff nurse may ponder on whether the ward team disintegrates when she is on leave. If it does, then the style of leadership may have something to do with it.

3.7. Positive behaviours in groups

Individuals involved in any form of working or learning group tend to display certain positive behaviours. These behaviours can be of two types. The first set of behaviours helps to get the task in hand effectively completed. For example some individuals in the group may contribute fresh ideas to help enrich the task in hand. The second set of behaviours helps the group to function effectively in terms of its dynamics. For example, some individuals may show enthusiasm and support other people's ideas.

Some members may show more initiative than others, and start discussions off; and if discussions stall for any reason, these individuals can breathe new life into them. The discussion may be steered into a new direction, or a new perspective on the issue being discussed may be gleaned. In short, some members tend to be more proactive than others. This is important because interest in issues can wane, and therefore the more proactive members have a useful role to play.

Group work and discussions can get stale and 'heavy'. Therefore, humour and 'looking at the funny side of things' is of value in group situations. The 'joker' in the group provides relief, and the group has time to unload briefly the weighty issue being discussed. Humour provides breathing space. It must be controlled, however; too much humour can imbalance the amount of time and effort spent on the task in hand.

Whereas some members may be over-talkative, others may be too quiet for comfort, and they will only contribute sporadically. They seem to take a back seat preferring to observe what is going on, and being said. These individuals must not be dismissed as uninterested, as they tend to observe on the direction the discussion is taking. They then try to put the discussion on course again. Observers tend to be reactive, and they have an important role in extending and enriching ideas produced by others. The observer may also summarize what has been achieved up to a point, and establish a new base from which the discussion can take off.

Some members can be perceived as a threat to the dynamics of a group because they are forever questioning or asking for extra information. It is easy to perceive these individuals as negative and of no value to the group. However, at the very least, it is a sign that interest is not waning. Questioners challenge assumptions made by group members. They also question shaky arguments and ask members to clarify unclear statements and generalizations. This puts pressure on the group members to be specific and clear about the issue in hand.

In a settled and mature group, members feel secure as there is trust and understanding. When the group has reached such a state, some individuals will contribute personal experiences that relate to the task in hand or issue being discussed. This helps to give the deliberations a certain amount of personal flavour. In addition, the extra information contributed may be of value to the task in hand. Contributions from such sources extend and enrich the group's task.

The above are positive behaviours, and may help the group in two ways. Firstly, they help to oil the machinery of the group, in that they make the flow of discussions easier. Secondly, they help in extending and enriching the deliberation or task in hand, whether it relates to a work group or a teaching group. Members also change roles during sessions. The joker may turn observer or questioner. The group leader needs to be aware of these positive behaviours, and to be able to use them to get the best out of either a learning or a work group.

3.8. Negative behaviours in groups

Positive behaviours, as looked at in the previous section, help to enhance the tasks and processes of groups. There are some behaviours, however, that can disrupt the tasks and processes of groups. Some individuals may have legitimate reasons for feeling under-used and uninvolved in some group sessions. Some may feel insecure for various reasons. Such members may react by being over-critical, appear uninterested, sidestep issues, and generally cause disruption. Behaviours such as these challenge the authority and respect the leader may have. If such behaviours are not handled effectively, they may sour the dynamics of sessions, and misdirect and confuse the group in terms of its objectives.

Individuals who are over-critical, either overtly or covertly, may be unclear about the objectives of the group, or may not have grasped the intricacies of the issues being dealt with. They may also be feeling uninvolved and on the periphery of the group. The leader, if faced with such a situation, may avoid being defensive, and try to reclarify the roles of individuals and the objectives of the sessions. He may listen to the reasons for the criticisms levelled, and if justified, acknowledge the critical contribution as a positive way of dealing with such a situation.

Some members may challenge another member's status, often

the leader's. Challenging another member's status may be a sign of insecurity. If faced with such a situation, one strategy for the leader to use is to build on the support that may be forthcoming from other members. Skilled members will often come to the rescue of the leader. It is also important to bear in mind that dissenters frustrate the dynamics and the task of the group. It may, therefore, be wise to leave other group members to confront challengers. If all else fails, disruptive members may be given the option of leaving the group, either for a particular session or for good.

Cliques may evolve in groups. Like-minded members may loosely identify with each other, and have a spokesperson or a sub-leader. These sub-groups may evolve a life of their own, and eventually may threaten the entity of the group. However, in most cases, clique formation is a natural development in group dynamics. At times some cliques exist on the peripheries of groups, and their contribution may be either negative or nonexistent. If such a situation exists, the leader may divide and distribute the task among the different members in the group, and plan to reconvene at a later date. Usually, at the reconvention, the dynamics within the cliques will have weakened or changed.

3.9. Conclusion

Groups go through set patterns of development and maturity. They offer potential in terms of the richness of experiences members bring to sessions. This potential is of immense importance to group leaders. The leaders can tap the experiences of the group and make teaching and learning more student-centered, the leader being the facilitator in the process. The group leader may use the experiences and expertise within the group to achieve the group's aims. The skilled leader will 'ride round' negative behaviours and build on positive behaviours and support. The outcome can be surprising!

References

Festinger, L. *et al.* (1963) *Social pressures in informal groups*, Tavistock.

Tuckman, B. (1973) in Napier, R.W., Gerfhenfeld, M.K. (eds) *Group Theory and Experience*, Houghton Mifflin, Boston.

White, R. and Lippitt, R. (1960) *Autocracy and democracy*, Harper and Row, New York.

Further reading

Fontana, D. (1988) *Psychology for Teachers*, 2nd edn British Psychological Association, London.

Hand, L. (1981) *Nursing Supervision*, Reston Publishing Co., Inc., Virginia.

Jackson, P.W. (1967) *Life in Classrooms*, Holt, Rinehart and Winston, New York.

Morrison, A. and MacIntyre, D. (1973) *Teachers and Teaching*, 2nd Ed., Penguin, Harmondsworth.

Payne, M. (1982) *Working in Teams*, Macmillan, London.

Sherif, M. (1936) *The Psychology of Social Norms*, Harper, New York.

Walton, M. (1984) *Management and Managing – A dynamic approach*, Harper and Row, London.

Yablonsky, L. (1967) *The Violent Gang*, Penguin, Harmondsworth.

4

Teaching in clinical areas

Jim Reid

teach, *tech,* v.t. to show: to direct: to impart knowledge or art to: to guide the studies of: to exhibit so as to impress upon the mind: to impart the knowledge or art of: to accustom: to counsel.

Chambers Twentieth Century Dictionary, Revised edition

Not only is there an art in teaching a thing,
but also a certain art in teaching it.

Cicero, De Legibus

4.1. Introduction

It would appear from the first definition that teaching, with its variety of meanings, is an activity impossible for anyone to avoid doing. The quotation coming from the ancient Roman orator Cicero tells us that people have been doing it for a very long time. In modern times this ancient 'art' is commonly referred to as being the sole activity of certain kinds of people called 'teachers' in certain kinds of places called 'schools'. This extremely confined view of the subject fails to recognize the real diversity of teachers around. Each of us in our own way has encountered the most unexpected of teachers who have taught us some new facet of the world; the baby who helped its mother to mother, an eight-year-old who instructed her budgie to make pert remarks, even the dead continue to teach us something about the world! The list is endless. It seems that teaching is a product of being alive – you cannot help doing it. Conscious or incognisant, you **will** teach. The staff nurse is no exception, whatever she may think. If there is any problem about teaching it will be about the 'certain' art.

There are quite obvious teaching functions and responsibilities within the overall role of the staff nurse. Whatever the different specialisms, skills, client-groups, backgrounds and backdrops the staff nurse works from, each is obliged to implicate teaching as a fundamental part of her professional life and work. This obligation is not restricted to student nurses and patients, but towards relatives, doctors, porters, administrators and any others who require nursing information.

The subject of teaching/teachers is huge. Countless volumes have been and no doubt will continue to be written about it. The subject receives the attention of all and sundry, from lollypop licking truants to university professors. It is analysed from a variety of points of view including philosophy, sociology, psychology, politics, etc. One wonders what else can be written that isn't a reinvention of the wheel! The teaching of nursing does not require any new rules that are not already established in the theory of education. The teaching environment of nursing is well documented in Ogier (1987), Alexander (1983) and Quin (1988), for example. The nature of nursing itself may still require investigation and sorting out and this will no doubt present teaching problems. However it is not the purpose of this chapter to define what nursing is.

Our aim is to try to make this universal activity interesting for the reader. The choice of themes are those we consider worthy of a teacher who gives some thought to it.

For those who wish to study a particular aspect of teaching, reference should be made to the appropriate specialist texts.

For the purposes of this chapter we use the staff-student nurse context and relationship. It would be too cumbersome and complicated to have to keep referring to others. However, it is usual to find points in a discussion on teaching which have general application whatever the context.

4.2. The teacher's pet

The teacher needs to have a student. To help understand what the teacher is and what she does, we need to have some idea about the nature of the person she is going to teach.

The term 'teacher's pet' may be a useful starting point as it is frequently quoted as the archetypal student. There are at least two possible interpretations of the term: that he is a preeny character who is the first to raise his hand, gives the correct answers, writes 'excellent' essays, never speaks the brogue, and wears polished Clark shoes. He is the apple of the teacher's eye. The other possible interpretation is that he is some sort of wild beast who is to be trained, tamed and chained into becoming some ideal type desired of by his headmaster.

These two student types may possibly exist. If they do, are they typical of all students, or are they parodies of the contradictions that exist in the nature of all students? Are students torn between willing and wanting to 'learn' whilst retaining some force resisting 'learning'? If learning implies 'change in the behaviour' it seems reasonable to presume that learning is sometimes desired and sometimes opposed. This phenomenon is frequently observed in ourselves and others: e.g., a belief that man has evolved from an hominid ancestry is opposed by a belief in his creationist origin; the use of 'models of nursing' is considered as idling badinage emanating from the occupants of the Ivory Tower; the widow who denies the reality of her husband's death.

One could go on for ever quoting examples clearly demonstrating the existence of these contrary and seemingly antagonistic forces. How and why they come into effect in an individual at a particular time would entail a massive study of the human sciences which only a Toynbee could attempt with any degree of success. Instead of seeing these paired forces as always being in opposition to each other, they might in fact be an essential intrapersonal precondition for learning to occur at all! In practice it might explain why we have a tendency to ask questions.

The student then would seem to be a collective contradiction with tendencies to destroy and construct. The teacher is wise to know him well. Three student features seem especially important for our understanding of him.

The student wants to learn. He is motivated and ready. The substance of each individual's motivation will vary in kind and degree. To one particular person it is to achieve a good reputation, whatever the cost; to another it is the satisfaction of discovery. The stimulus to arousal states varies from individual to individual and from time to time. It is not always under the person's control nor of his own choosing. Many factors in his environment, internal and external, will have some influence on motivation. The teacher, as the stimulus, may not always invoke a favourable reaction. She has to consider her own motivations towards the student, which may or may not match his needs.

Readiness refers to our ability and capability to respond. It is what is implied when we say that the child will walk when he is 'ready' to walk. This readiness to walk acts on him to want to walk – it is a precursor to motivation.

Readiness represents the condition and preparedness of the organism (e.g., the student) to make and decide its next move. This 'next move' potential is derived and conduced from the predisposition available in the organism's physical and mental set. Learning is the 'next move' instituting a change in these two sets, which, being changed, create a new condition for learning. The limits to learning are not known. Professor C.H. Waddington (1977) writes that 'My guess – it can be no more than a guess – is that no one – Einstein, Plato, Leonardo – has ever yet had the opportunity to develop his mental genetic program to the point where it reaches termination and sets a limit on his capacities.' What **is** learned however is another matter. The implications for the student and teacher are profound.

Let's suppose a staff nurse teaches a student the method of injecting a drug intramuscularly – the student has never done this before. She teaches him in the manner she knows how to, and the student duly learns her method. He later considers himself able and capable of administrating an intramuscular injection. On examination by his charge nurse supervisor he is found to be making errors of commission and omission. (The actual mistakes are not important for the analogy, they are of course ominous in the real situation.) The student is surprised. The charge nurse asks him to explain his mistakes. He replies, 'It was how I was taught!' (A not uncommon exculpatory explanation which shows up two processes, firstly, when is the student entitled to be responsible and secondly, where does the fault lie, in the method or in the 'thing' taught?)

Give both the student and the teacher the benefit of innocence and our charitableness; nevertheless, what conditions might have resulted in his incomplete and mistaken abilities? The following may have been involved.

1. Errors not identified or rectified.
2. Incomplete learning.
3. Lack of referential indices.
4. Inadequate supervision.
5. Insufficient practice.
6. Disjunctions between the task and goals ('He won't feel a thing, it's only a jab!')

7. Incompatibilities between the student and his teacher.
8. Interferences.

These are some of the conditions where control has been lost by the teacher. Sometimes the environment of nursing creates these conditions for student and teacher. However we can't be absolved from all responsibility as the consequences are far-reaching. Supposing the student's bad practice and misunderstanding had continued unabated, his way of doing it would become established as normative. If, at a much later date, the errors of his way are revealed to him, he would then be faced with at least three problems; to unlearn a set pattern of interlinked behaviours, to learn new substitute behaviours, and to conquer disharmonious feelings, thoughts, attitudes etc. This would involve the expenditure of a lot of energy which he might not find easy to spare. This consequential process is increased if the skill, wrongly learned, is of a greater magnitude.

Lastly but of similar importance is the question of dealing with individual differences (Remington and Kroll, 1990). Does the student learn only what is pre-ordained by the syllabus or can he decide his own progress within the syllabus according to his own learning needs? As learning contains its own momentum and restraints, students who are inadequately or insufficiently stimulated by the educational system will divert their energies outside the system or outside the controls of the system. Examples of the former could include such activities as intense socializing, joining karate clubs, planning for the holiday to Greece next year. Examples of the latter might include the student attempting to initiate some aspect of professional practice for which he is not prepared, or to assume competence based on non-curricular criteria such as status, personal experience, or boredom.

The student only wants to learn after all!

Students want to be skilled practitioners. Whether it is as basic as learning to walk or as sophisticated as a Paganini capriccio, the desire of the performer is to achieve the action(s) commensurate with the nature and form of the activity. The activity therefore has to be defined and measurable according to some quantitative and qualitative standard if it is to become realized. The activity of nursing, which is really a rubric for a concatenation of certain prescribed activities, has to demonstrate structure, form and rules for it to function logically. If these are absent then the activity is just driftwood in a sea of tall ships.

Skill is the ability to perform the activity defined. To become skilled will entail the student undergoing a series of patterned changes to existing knowledge adaptive to the contingencies of the activity. This is not just a mechanical process producing a machine-like operation – the skilled person isn't a robot that has 'learnt' (mimicked is a more accurate term) to walk or fiddle. The missing factor in the machine which is inherent in the person, is, *mutatis mutandis*, the aesthetic with its principles of sensitivity, harmony, poise, and beauty. Skill combines technique and art. There is no compromise.

How then can the teacher help him to become a 'skilled practitioner'? At first sight the answer seems obvious – bring out the *Manual of Nursing Procedures*, open at the relevant page, point to the activity, note its procedural composition, show him the means, tell him to 'watch me' carefully, instruct him in the rites of passage, and expect to hear a sonorous duet echo down the hospital corridor!

There is nothing much wrong with this ordered approach as far as it goes, and in the hands of a 'good' teacher and a 'clever' student it could conceivably succeed, though only if certain conditions are being met.

1. The manual is from the nursing body of knowledge.
2. The teacher is a nurse.
3. The activity is a nursing activity.
4. The teaching method contains opportunities to practise, regulated by a system of appraisal.

This last point has the most direct impact on the skill-learning process. Without it the student and teacher have no way of knowing how he is doing.

Opportunity to practise is a self-evident condition for learning and for maintaining that learning. The more opportunities available, the greater the likelihood of the skill being realized. During the process of skill-learning, the student will experience 'slip-ups' associated with the problem of integrating all the various elements into a coherent, smooth action. This network of integration takes time (depending on the degree of difficulty of the activity in question). The student needs opportunities to 'smooth out' or iron out these difficulties. He is further helped by the inclusion of a supporting appraisal system.

The essence of any appraisal system is feedback. This cybernetic principle helps to correct, regulate, and steady the state of the student. The student himself can generate his own feedback, either by methodically comparing himself with a desired standard, or intuitively judging his performance against it. Self-appraisal tends to predominate as we become more experienced, until a new set of circumstances occurs which requires an external source of feedback (e.g., from his teacher).

The importance of the teacher as expert, functioning as the source of feedback, cannot be underestimated or surrendered away. In the case of nursing, the teacher has an additional responsibility besides that of ensuring the integrity of the activity and student learning, she has also to ensure that obligations towards the patient are satisfied throughout.

Feedback from the teacher can come in two ways; as an exponent of the activity and as coach to the student. The student benefits most when the feedback is presented unambiguously and is directed at the behaviour in relation to the activity. Points of strength as well as weaknesses should be identified. This helps him to differentiate and distinguish each phase or pattern in the skill. It should be noted that this cybernetic feature of learning is not always easy or pleasant. In some ways, the term 'trial by ordeal' indicates what has at times to be experienced by both student and teacher!

Finally there is the moment of truth. If the patient expresses gratitude for a task well done, what better source of feedback to conclude that all the 'sweat and toil' has been worth it?

The student will have barriers to learning.

1. He pleads to play football as his mother tries to teach him how to tie his shoe laces.
2. He dreams of his 'Juliet' as the teacher declaims Romeo's infatuation.
3. His new shoes torture his heels as the charge nurse describes the technique of cardio-pulmonary resuscitation.
4. He clutches his crucifix as the lecturer asserts Darwinism.

Sometimes the student wants to learn but is unable to. Sometimes he is able to, but does not want to learn. If these curious contradictions reveal anything they prove the fallacy in the *tabula rasa* notion that learning is just a piling-up of one new fact upon another in the construction of a human termite-hill. As the cursory examples of 'anti-learning' above indicate, learning cannot be taken for granted, nor do the teacher and student always walk hand-in-hand. Barriers will and do exist to block learning; some are piddling coincidental events which are quickly passing and the student is able later to catch up. Some barriers are much more serious. What are those barriers? How do they affect learning? What can the student and teacher do about it?

As has already been stated, learning is a change of behaviour that involves energy. It seems reasonable to assume therefore that something can sometimes cause a bifurcation of the energy input and the change-of-behaviour output, so that the student who wants to learn can't, or the student who doesn't want to learn won't. That 'something' is the barrier. It may be tangible and distinctive such as a physical illness, a mental illness, family commitments, economic strains etc. Others can be more subtly intrusive, such as low self-esteem, embarrassment, fear, interpersonal rivalries, etc.

The student can be aware of the source and nature of the barrier(s) but for the moment is not able to circumvent or cope by alternative means. There is not much he can do if he is laid low with glandular fever, or phobic anxiety, or divorce of his parents.

Conversely the student is not aware of the source or nature of the barrier(s). He may not be able to admit that he has feelings of love/hatred towards his teacher (not unusual!), he may feel threatened by some idea which challenges a deeply held belief or value, he may not like the field of study but for some reason he feels compelled to stay.

These are just some of the many possible barriers to learning. They can have their origins in the student's own personal and social background unrelated to his professional training. However the barriers are frequently connected with some factors in the educational environment – nursing is redolent with them, e.g., exposure to cross infections, excessive physical and emotional loads, death, suffering, authoritarianism, irregular work patterns, violence, electroconvulsive therapy, abortion, etc. The student's exposure to these experiences will vary in intensity and duration. Many of them are unavoidable. His reactions will be brought into the learning situation.

To continue to teach anything to the student as if nothing is wrong is wasting time and energy. The throughput information will not be received, or will be received incompletely. All his cognitive processes will be those of the 'scattered-brain'; his memory, attention, concentration, perception, motivation, and emotions juxtaposed with his preoccupations with conflicting demands in his conscious and unconscious mind. He will at times indicate obvious signs of conflict; crying, fainting, lip-biting, muscle tremor, unpunctuality, clumsiness etc. Other signs are more elusive, such as conforming obedience, subtle facial movements – the furtive grin, quickly raised eyeborws, the puckered lips, the quick turn away etc.

It is hardly worth saying that the responsibility of the teacher now focuses on the condition of the student. This banal statement masks a potentially different order of business for the teacher. She may be confronted by a student who has erected a barrier as his only way, rightly or wrongly, to protect the integrity of his beliefs against the provocative challenge of her teachings.

4.3. The teacher's pet subject

I hear and forget.
I see and I remember.
I do and I know.

What does the teacher teach? On wearing her 'mortar-board' she says to the student that, 'Counselling is a part of the nursing role . . . etc. . . . ' What could the student make of that? What is she teaching? Is the student making the same sense of 'it' as she is? What has he possibly learnt? What was the teacher's intention?

Using the introductory aphorism and assuming that the student is in the best of all possible conditions for learning, let us see some possible learning outcomes.

The student sits behind a desk and listens attentively, occasionally writing down notes. The teacher speaks on-and-off for about an hour. Several hours later his friend asks him to recall the session. 'Well,' he begins, 'she talked about counselling, and went on about some American chap called Roy Rogers, I think, how we should ahem, regard unconcernedly the client's problems without judging them worthless. And she said that sick people don't want counselling from anyone but someone who ahem, they fancy. Know what I mean? Anyhow she sounded keen on the subject. Oh yes, she gave us a handout at the end.'

His friend then asks him to describe the teacher. 'Well,' taking a deep breath, 'She was, I would say about 40, wore tinted glasses, and really fiery red lipstick. She wore a polka-dot cravat over a white collar. Not bad looking either. Had on a blue suit. She sat in front of the class. Nice-looking legs, certainly didn't have varicose veins. She spoke Morningside patois, very lah-di-dah. Oh, and she didn't have any rings on.'

Finally his friend asks him if he knows how to counsel. 'Counsel!' he exclaims, 'Me counsel! You must be joking. I wouldn't know where to start.'

It would appear from this not untypical cartoon sketch that we can postulate several important points about learning and teaching.

The teacher and the message are two different kinds of information to the student. The strength of one over the other will attract the focus of his attention. In this case her appearance is more attractive than her spoken message – her visual signals (lipstick, legs, spectacles, etc.) dominate her oratorical ones from the student's point of view at the time.

The language in her oral message contain elements which are understood and others which are not understood. The nominal term, Carl Rogers, was later recalled mistakenly as Roy Rogers. The mistake could be related either to difficulties in the reception, retention or recall of information. These functions of memory are strained by pre- and coexisting information circumventing the new information having to be dealt with by the student. The possible derivatory factors behind this particular fault of memory, i.e., inaccurate recall of 'Carl Rogers' could lie in its close literal association with the American film star-cum-cowboy Roy Rogers, or the American 'Roy adaptation model' of nursing, both being familiar to the student than was the prenominal 'Carl'.

The teacher and the student will always have the problem of understanding and memorizing new data accurately. Nursing, like all other specialized activities, has a preponderance of recondite terminology which the uninitiated find both formidable and intriguing but the initiated take for granted.

The teacher and the message are indivisible in that the message contains qualities as projected in the teacher's para-lingual exposition. Put simply, if the teacher voices enthusiasm and belief in 'counselling' it will at that point appear to the student a convincing subject to be interested in. Conversely, if she projects undertones of boredom and doubt, this may be read as representing the nature of the subject. 'The sound must seem an echo to the sense' (Pope).

The teacher and the student are two separate ontological entities with different levels of experience. If the teacher treats the student as a standard entity, without individuality, she can never ascertain his covalancy with her intentions in her teaching. She might as well be a tape recorder, which at least allows the student to control the on-off switch according to the dictates of the occasion.

The teacher and the student are a 'dynamic duo'. This batmanesque relationship succinctly defines that state of partnership and interaction played out in the 'classroom'. How they relate with each other may or may not be conducive to the needs of either or both. A relationship of congeniality and mutual respect around the common purpose of learning is considered an essential foundation for learning from each other. To behave rigidly according to a form of stereotype casting, i.e., the teacher dominates and the student submits, will tend to teach aspects of a 'hidden curriculum' (discussed below) rather than the objective of the 'lesson' (e.g., counselling) which brought them together in the first place.

The teacher teaches 'counselling'; why? And by teaching counselling what else is she teaching?

The usual answer to the first question is that counselling (and other subjects) is taught because it is in the curriculum. The unusual answer to the second question is that counselling (like the other subjects) is taught by the 'hidden curriculum'. Curriculum and its incubus brother Hidden need to be defined!

According to Nichols and Nichols (1978): 'Curriculum is all the opportunities planned by teachers for pupils.'

In her essay, 'Some Aspects of The Hidden Curriculum' (1987), Margaret Pearl Treacy quotes Jenkins and Shipman as suggesting that the hidden curriculum 'includes all those pervasive values that one is expected to acquire by a process of institutional seepage; things like punctuality, good behaviour, tolerance of frustration, loyalty. These and other influences on the individual come from his or her involvement in an organization with consistent assumptions as well as specific objectives, an elaborate set of expectations as well as a specific mode of working. Over time, traditions and rituals are developed which reinforce the influence exerted over the individual.' Later in the same essay Treacy herself writes that, 'The hidden curriculum is encountered not just in the classroom but also in the clinical areas of hospital wards and departments.'

To the individual teacher this means that she is a spoke in a wheel, only one of many other influences acting on the student. The final outcome, when the student becomes a qualified nurse, will bear only some resemblance to those planned outcomes as asserted in the official curriculum. Nursing and nurse are two quite different states, nursing being an ideal type, whereas the nurse is a social type. Nursing is what links nurses, and differentiates them from other types in the same way as doctors and medicine, historians and history, poets and poetry. The hidden curriculum through its 'pervasive' influence 'makes' the nurse.

To the extent that counselling becomes a function of the nurse, it will mainly be confirmed if it is experienced 'pervasively'. Counselling has to compete with other nursing functions such as wound care, technological applications, chemotherapeutics, etc. The staff nurse may mention or even teach counselling, but if her nurse practice excludes counselling, significantly because of other chosen priorities, then the disparity will tend to diminish the importance of counselling as a necessary nurse activity. The message in the hidden curriculum is that other nursing activities are paramount.

To the extent that counselling **is** pervasive, suggesting therefore that it is a routine function of the nurse does not necessarily mean that counselling is being practised according to its ideal type. If the student is 'counselled' and in the course of which he is told 'to pull his socks up!' then counselling is associated with a form of disciplining. If this association is maintained long enough, then counselling is perceived as an administrative procedure. Also, if counselling is prescribed for the patient to be given by a qualified counsellor, then the subject is seen as the work for experts in the technique, not for the generic nurse – let alone the student nurse.

To ignore the hidden curriculum, the teacher perforce is fooling herself if she believes the content and method of her teaching is instrumental in the formation of the student-becoming-a-nurse. Somehow the teacher has to ensure as little disparity as possible between these curricula, lest the actual learning outcomes become inimical to those desired. One consequence of this unevenness leads to the student experiencing such a state of **cognitive dissonance** to cause him to leave nursing permanently, or end up practising nursing according to some parochial conventionality. To reduce this possibility, the staff nurse as teacher must *ipso facto* be included in the design, implementation and evaluation processes of curriculum development.

The teacher's 'pet subject' may only wag its tail at her!

4.4. What's your teacher's name – Anathema Sit?

After 'my mother' and 'my father', the next most important figure in the history of an individual is 'my teacher'. As I wrote in my introduction, the teacher is potentially anyone of any age and description, and is not limited to those labelled as 'teacher'. This raises some intriguing issues. Firstly, no one can deny or reject this entitlement since their actions, unbeknown to themselves might be internalized into another person's domain. Secondly, the universality of the teaching-effect forces us to acknowledge the immeasurability of some kinds of learning that are constantly occurring beyond our conscious awareness. This is both reassuring and unsettling. It is reassuring in the sense that ordinary, everyday human transactions maintain and generate existential wisdom to counterbalance the doctrines of formal scholasticism. It is unsettling in that answering the question, 'What have you learnt?', the respondant will only be able to answer what he thinks he has learned, not what he knows he has learned, which is impossible. And so the debates and arguments will continue forever.

What is not in dispute is the undisguised teacher. For better or for worse these figures mark their ticks and crosses on our efforts and imaginations.

In our infancy she is a cherubic giant, smiling under her halo, or a monstrous gargoyle belching forth the furies. Her image sticks to the skin like scar tissue. In adolescence he sees her as a fool who scratches herself whilst giggling at her own jokes. In mature years she is a rare inspiration, perchance met along the way. As indicated at the beginning of this essay, she can be found sucking her dummy while fumbling in domestic detritus inventing objects out of shoe boxes; she is the precocious youth making the seemingly impossible become possible; she is the dead one whose legacy in print, canvas or sound cause him surprised awakening.

Teachers come and go in all sorts of guises; she may wear smart clothes, she may smoke, she may be an academic, she may be a singer of songs. Whoever she is, she is You! Someone will have your image adhering to their skin.

In recent times the old term 'teacher' has come under a barrage of competing substitutes. Curious names like mentor, buddy, preceptor, guru, facilitator and supervisor are just a few of these challenging titles.

Advocates of one or other of these synonymous terms will no doubt reason out and carefully describe their chosen favourite. Whether they provide an easier path to the art of teaching with its variety of forms, its quest for exactitude, its unending debates, etc. is questionable. Their fanciful look seem brittle against the teachings of the teacher.

What is more important than these singularly interesting nominations is the relationship between teaching and learning, and between teacher and student. Hopefully neither one will name the other as *anathema sit* (let him be accursed).

References

1. Alexander, M. (1983) *Learning to be a Nurse*, Churchill Livingstone, Edinburgh.
2. Nichols, A. and Nichols, H. (1978) *Developing a Curriculum* (2nd edn), Allen and Unwin, London.
3. Ogier, M. (1982) *An Ideal Sister*, RCN, London.
4. Ogier, M. (1987) *The Learning Environment in Clinical Nursing*, Scutari Projects Ltd, Harrow on the Hill, Middlesex.
5. Quin, F.M. (1988) *Principles and Practice of Nurse Education*, (2nd Ed.), Croom Helm, London.
6. Remington, M.A., and Kroll, C. (1990) The High-Risk Nursing Student: Identifying the characteristics and learning style preferences, *Nurse Education Today*, Feb., 10: 1.
7. Treacy, M.P., (1987) Some Aspects of the Hidden Curriculum, in *The Curriculum in Nursing Education*, Allan, P. and Jolley, M. (eds.), Croom Helm, London.
8. Waddington, C.H., (1977) *Tools for Thought*, Paladin, London.

5

Assessment of students

Stanley Walker

5.1. Assessment

The assessment of staff is an area which most individuals find difficult because of the very personal nature of the task. The ability to assess successfully requires an understanding of the basic philosophy and principles of assessment, and can involve a considerable re-learning process. There is no short cut to being able to think objectively, and this may require some experimentation.

5.5.1. Assessing students

Assessment of students must be regarded as a serious responsibility, as the collective outcome of such assessments will determine whether or not the student is considered to be a person who can be recommended to the United Kingdom Central Council.

The basic principles underlying the process of student and pupil nurse assessment are set out below and can be applied to any type of documentation or reporting system in use.

What is Assessment?

The purpose of the assessment is to provide supervisors and teachers with a clear picture of the student throughout training. It helps to make and keep the student aware of her progress and enables her to participate in her own assessment.

Assessment, therefore, should be a continuous process in which the learner and the assessors are equally involved. It is important to appreciate that any completed assessment should present a clear picture of either lack of progress or improvement in performance throughout a period of clinical experience.

5.1.2. Who assesses?

Satisfactory assessment is essentially a team activity, involving the ward sister, staff nurse, teaching staff and the student. The various members of the team approach the subject from different angles but collectively contribute to the total assessment.

Recognizing pitfalls

The difficulty of setting a standard against which to judge students is a problem which must be resolved before any assessment is undertaken. It is easy to say that a student is 'average', but what comparison can be used? A student can be compared with other students in her particular intake; this most certainly results in a great variety of standards.

Alternatively, she can be assessed against what can reasonably be expected of a student at that particular stage in training. The difficulty here is that different assessors have different ideas of what can be expected of students.

There is no easy solution to this problem, but it is suggested that regular discussions between clinical staff and teachers could do much to smooth over such differences and produce a more even standard. Also, having defined learning objectives for the period of clinical allocation will ensure that each student is assessed on the ability to achieve these objectives.

Failure to maintain a fair perspective

A certain episode or episodes in the student's time in a clinical area can be imprinted on the assessor's mind and, if taken in isolation, can give a false impression of the student's overall performance, either to the advantage or disadvantage of the student. For example, the student may have acted in a commendable manner in an emergency situation or, on the other hand, may have made an error of judgement in carrying out a procedure.

In such cases, it is helpful to keep a note of these incidents provided that the incidents are freely discussed with the student.

Interpersonal relationships can also have a strong effect on assessment of one person by another. You should always aim for objectivity in order to present a balanced opinion. Failure to appreciate that people, too often unconsciously and unreasonably, associate certain levels of achievement with certain physical characteristics, outward appearance, or manner, may influence an assessment.

Objectivity can be reduced by failing to appreciate that the assessor's own clinical area is a new experience for each student. It is sometimes easy to assume that the level of knowledge of all the students in the same area is equal. Allowances should be made for the length of time the student has been in training.

The result may also be affected by how the assessor feels, both physically and mentally. A second review after a lapse of twenty-four to forty-eight hours under different circumstances helps to ensure maximum objectivity. A review on the same lines by another member of the assessing team is an added safeguard.

In addition it is important to appreciate the possible adverse effects of unusual circumstances, such as staff shortages, or some unexpected crisis during the period over which the assessment is being made. It is equally important that the student should be kept informed of the results of any review of an assessment she has previously discussed.

5.2. The process of assessment

5.2.1. First requirements

In order to produce a good assessment of the student, both learner (student) and assessor (trained nurse) have certain requirements which must be met.

The assessor requires information regarding the following aspects.

1. The course curriculum.
2. Any previous training undertaken by the student, e.g., training in another discipline.
3. The stage of training reached by the student.
4. Details of the student's practical experience.
5. What clinical objectives have previously been achieved.
6. What clinical objectives have to be achieved during this experience.

This information can be acquired from the student and the college or school of nursing.

Further important information can be obtained only from the student, such as the following.

1. The student's own view of her training needs.

2. The student's attitude to previous training in other clinical areas.

On her side the student needs to know the following.

1. The type and nature of nursing carried out in the ward.
2. The experience she can hope to achieve during this placement.
3. Her personal responsibilities in the ward environment.

5.2.2. Preliminary interview

Trained nurses are increasingly conscious that a brief informal discussion with the student at the beginning of the placement is of mutual benefit. Orientation to the ward is also beneficial in familiarizing the student with the patients, staff and ward layout.

Pressure of work should not prevent this preliminary interview becoming an essential part of the assessment process for all students. It may be useful to examine the pattern of work in the ward to determine ways and means of making such an interview an integral part of that pattern.

Ideally this should take place in a relaxed atmosphere where the assessor and student can be free from interruptions. It should not be a session of 'dos' and 'don'ts', but rather an exploration by both parties when the 'first requirements' mentioned above can be checked and discussed. If a good rapport can be established, it should be possible for the trained nurse to identify some of the individual problems of the student, on which special guidance and instruction may be needed. In this respect it would be useful for the assessor to make some notes on any relevant points which can be used when reviewing the student's performance at a later date.

5.2.3. Continuous assessment

The completion of an assessment report is only the final act of a continuous process. The preliminary interview should produce some kind of initial assessment of the student to serve as a basis from which to work.

It is vitally important that each assessor should be as objective as possible in reviewing the student's progress. For this reason, it is not advisable for previous assessments to be forwarded from one assessor to the next, as it is only too easy to be influenced by the comments of others, or even by the hospital grapevine, and thus start with a biased or prejudiced view.

Progressive assessment should therefore take the form of observing the student's work and attitude to work, teaching by direct questioning and regular discussion of the student's work with her on a regular basis. In assessing skills the assessor should remember to assess not only the skill but also the underlying knowledge and attitudes in carrying out that skill. It is accepted that assessing attitude may be a difficult area to assess as acceptable attitudes are very personal and individualistic qualities. Nevertheless, the assessor must make a judgement based on whether the nurse's attitude would be acceptable to the client, i.e., the patient, or his or her relatives.

The basic principles underlying continuous assessment should be that faults are pointed out to the student when they occur and steps should be taken to overcome them. It is wrong to allow the learner to drift along in the mistaken belief that she is giving satisfaction when this is not so.

Commendation on work well done is just as important as the correction of faults. The psychological effect of a word of praise can hardly be overestimated.

5.2.4. Student self-assessment

It has been found that students asked to assess their own work are frequently more critical of themselves than other assessors. To encourage learners to acquire a constantly critical attitude to their progress and performance is helpful in teaching self accountability, and students should be encouraged to do this from the outset of their training. Students should also be asked to identify positive aspects of their performance so that their confidence is maintained.

5.3. Writing the assessment

The emphasis should always be on accurately measuring the student's progress over the period of the clinical placement, and should reflect both the student's contribution to patient care and whether or not she has achieved the learning objectives for this placement.

Although continuous assessment should be the aim, it is useful to carry out an interim assessment on several occasions. These give the assessor and the student the opportunity to identify strengths and weaknesses so that appropriate teaching and experience can be concentrated where most needed during subsequent experience.

The assessor will find it useful to make notes of the interim assessments as they will be helpful when writing the final assessment report.

When writing the final report it is important that the student should not be compared with others. The assessment should refer to progress and the quality of her work.

If assessors find themselves giving a greater proportion of high or low ratings then they should consider whether this results from one of two possible causes.

1. Having an unusually good or poor group of students.
2. A personal tendency to be lenient or harsh in her judgement of students.

If the assessors find themselves giving scarcely any ratings outside two or three grades, it is again necessary to consider whether this results from one of two possibilities.

1. Having a group which has much less variation than usual.
2. Reluctance to make reasonably marked distinctions in judgement of subordinates.

An answer giving (2) in either case indicates the need for a revision in the assessor's standard of judgement.

5.4. The assessment interview

A date and time should be arranged shortly before the student leaves the ward, to ensure reasonable conditions for a quiet discussion.

It is important that this interview should take place in a situation where both parties feel relaxed and able to concentrate on the task in hand. It is probably best to restrict the interview to the assessor and the student nurse alone, although the inclusion of another trained nurse may be useful, providing that the arrangement is acceptable to all concerned.

This interview should concentrate on a review of the student's work and progress since the preliminary interview, using the interim assessments as a guide. Many assessors may find it difficult to complete the assessment form in the presence of the student and would prefer to do so in private after full discussion. Whichever method is adopted, it is essential that each heading is discussed with the student who is given the opportunity to put her own point of view.

It is essential that the student should know exactly what has been written about her before the assessment is sent to the college or school of nursing.

Most assessment forms require the student to sign that she has read and understood the report though not necessarily agreeing with the contents. It is only fair, however, that if the student feels that she has good reason to disagree with anything in the report, she should have the right to put her own reasons and point of view in writing, and that her statement should accompany the report.

5.5. Writing the assessment report

This is undoubtedly the most difficult area of assessment for the inexperienced, and most assessors will need help and guidance when undertaking written reports until confidence has been gained in committing thoughts to paper.

Assessment forms vary considerably throughout the Health Service, and some are more helpful than others, depending on how the form is structured. Whatever form is used will nevertheless require the assessor to write comments on the student, and it is important to consider how your report will be interpreted by the person reading it.

The report should avoid the use of one-word comments such as excellent, good or average. It should be concise and use short but meaningful statements, which will give to the reader a clear picture of the student's performance. Try not to be too general, and use specific examples of how the student has functioned, e.g., 'gives clear instructions to juniors, and always checks understanding' is much better than saying 'has leadership qualities'.

Before committing herself to paper the assessor should consider the overall impression that she wishes to convey in the report. Try at this stage to make brief notes on the points you wish to make, and show these to other trained staff who have been involved in working with the student. Try also to determine whether the impressions you have are opinions or facts.

Remember that any weaknesses should be considered in view of the overall function of the student and the situation obtaining in the ward over the period of the assessment. You should also consider factors such as staffing levels, how busy the ward was, and any pesonal difficulties which the student may have had outside the working environment, such as sickness or family problems.

You should now be ready to write the assessment, but before you do you may find it useful to go over your brief notes once again, and discard any extraneous material or add additional comments which you feel have been missed.

Having written the report consider whether it gives a clear and accurate picture and is complete. If you feel that you have covered all aspects of the assessment, put the report aside for a day or two and read it again. If you are still satisfied with your comments then you have most probably written a fair and accurate assessment.

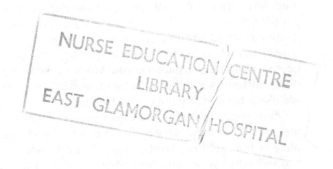

6

Problem counselling

Arthur Thwaites

6.1. Introduction

No doubt the area in which you are staffing will make a big difference to the amount of counselling you are already doing. Psychiatric, mental handicap and rehabilitation settings often set a high priority on nurses discussing problems with patients. This may also apply to staff nurses working in health centres or people's own homes. In contrast, some acute areas within general hospitals stress the urgent need to preserve life, and this may crowd out or at least postpone paying attention to emotional needs. However, wherever you work, if your duties as a staff nurse include speaking to patients and their relatives, then you are likely to be doing some counselling.

Other factors which affect the amount of counselling you offer may include staff shortages, the number of tasks you aim to complete within set time limits, your own estimate of your ability to counsel effectively, and your own stress load at any given time. (It is not easy to support someone else at a time when you are feeling upset and vulnerable yourself.)

Fears about counselling

Should you concern yourself with the fears and worries of others? Are you afraid of allowing patients to open up their worries and private misery to you in case you cannot solve their troubles? Are you afraid of making things worse? Are you in danger of becoming over-involved, unable to switch off when you go off duty?

Some counselling is unavoidable

The bad news is that, even though you may be trying to avoid counselling altogether, sometimes the need arises right in front of your eyes and, short of running away, you just cannot avoid it. So at the very least it pays to have a kind of first-aid kit of counselling skills. Think of all the times when you will be the only trained person coping with distressed people: times when there won't be a senior nurse, a doctor, a social worker or a psychologist in sight. In any case, you are likely to be the one whom the person knows best, and it is not by accident that he has chosen to tell you about the hurt and fear. The good news is that you can learn how to help people with psychological problems and yet take care of yourself as well.

Please do not underestimate your ability to give comfort and support when it is needed

The nurse is often the one who is best placed to deal with distress at the time it arises. By your timely intervention you may be able to prevent untold suffering and to hasten the recovery process. It is not as though we are novices in counselling. Throughout our lives we have already had experience of being with friends and family when they, and we, have been coping with distressing events. As nurses we have developed our sensitivity to suffering, and it is often the nurse who is the first one to notice when patients and relatives are emotionally upset, anxious, angry, euphoric, depressed or whatever.

When I talk about problem counselling I am not just talking about having a wee chat, giving advice, cheering someone up, or reassuring the patient. I am talking about sensing and listening out for emotional pain, tuning in to the expressed and the covert messages, and responding to the underlying feelings.

6.2. Separating problem counselling from allied skills

In this chapter we will be focussing on problem counselling as distinct from other helping strategies. In your work you will come across many different kinds of counselling, and some of them are featured by other contributors to this book. In this chapter we will concentrate on problem counselling exclusively, and that means that we will not be covering equally important skills like career counselling, disciplinary counselling, direct action (in which we ourselves take what we consider to be the most suitable action for someone else's needs), teaching (giving someone else the information which we think that they need in order to solve a problem), giving advice (telling someone what we think they should do, and how, when and where they should do it).

These all presuppose that we know what is best for someone, whereas in problem counselling we do not make such an assumption. There are many other types of helping strategies and psychotherapy too, but they are also beyond the scope of this chapter.

6.3. Definitions of problem counselling

We will begin by considering three definitions of problem counselling.

1. 'Helping someone to explore a problem so that they can decide what to do about it.' (I don't know who first said this, but I like its brevity.)
2. 'The task of counselling is to give the client an opportunity to explore, discover, and clarify ways of living more resourcefully and towards greater well being.' (Working Group of British Association of Counselling, B.A.C. 37a Sheep Street, Rugby (1982).)
3. 'Creating the sort of relationship within which a person can thrive and feel safe enough to face current difficulties in his/her life. This entails providing support whilst the person tries changing from old self-defeating ways to new more adaptive behaviour.' (Thwaites.)

I keep changing my definition as I respond to the needs of different people so the above is not immutable. Hopefully you will make your definitions too, because your aims in problem counselling will certainly affect the outcome. Something else which will affect the outcome is the sort of person you are yourself. *Ninety per cent of your potential effectiveness as a counsellor arises from the sort of person you are yourself, your own personal qualities and the way you interact with people.*

After you have read the next two paragraphs, please stop reading and do an exercise which will last for a full twenty minutes. The aim of this exercise is to highlight a list of qualities which you would like to find in an ideal counsellor.

To help you to focus in on this exercise, imagine that you personally have just had an awful succession of bad experiences and are looking for someone outside your family and close friends who can help you with all these calamities. If it is absolutely inconceivable to you that you would ever require a counsellor, then imagine that someone really close to you needs help for emotional problems and you are looking for the best counsellor there is.

Exercise 1. Write down a list of qualities which you would like to find in an ideal counsellor.

Though the exercise can be done by yourself alone, it is even better done in a small group of three or four people, so that you can share ideas and form a more comprehensive list. If the group contains people who are not nurses, there can be an advantage in that too. Please do give yourselve the full twenty minutes on this exercise before moving on to the next paragraph. It is crucial to what follows, and points us towards essential self-awareness. When you have completed this task, released your hijacked group members, and having given yourself a break, please take your time and read slowly through your list.

Exercise 2. Now read through the list again and mark the good counselling qualities which you yourself already possess.

You can either rate yourself straight off by using your self-knowl-edge, or, alternatively, you can imagine which qualities your pati-ents would say that you have. Be honest with yourself and don't underrate your good qualities. In fact I am going to ask you to look through the list again to see if you can't claim more of these good qualities for yourself. Don't be limited by the list either. There will be other good qualities which you can now recognize in yourself. Value these strengths. They are some of your best attributes, the bedrock of your ability to nurse, and when you are counselling allow these attributes to be clearly seen instead of hidden away. Making it that bit easier for a patient to relax and respond to you, can mean the difference between sharing a per-sonal problem, or worrying about it throughout the months ahead.

Exercise 3. Mark the good qualities which you don't really have in any appreciable degree, but which you might be able to foster.

In order to make any useful changes in your counselling qualities you will need to know what is going wrong. For example, I had not realized that I frowned ferociously when concentrating hard, and it wasn't until a colleague pointed this out to me (along with the effect it was having on clients) that I learned to change this. Likewise, for another example, it may be that you experience some difficulty in confronting constructively. Instead of leading to solutions the other person goes into defensive behaviour, denial, aggression, hurt feelings, crumbling, or whatever. Maybe you can learn to tackle such a situation in a more productive way as a result of analyzing recurring experiences in similar encounters. Or maybe you think that you could benefit from learning specific counselling skills designed to enlarge your repertoire when confronting and challenging.

Exercise 4. Mark the qualities of a good counsellor which you may despair of acquiring and/or qualities which you have no intention of acquiring.

In either case, paying attention to these feelings and respecting them is worthwhile. It may well be that these qualities are not for you, and trying to acquire them may make you feel false, unnatural, not genuine, and therefore non-effective. Sometimes it is a matter of having to accept blind spots in ourselves and, fortunately for all of us, there are usually ways of compensating for such gaps and still working effectively in our counselling. Certainly, counselling is not something to be done by numbers. (If he says A then I say B, and if he then jumps to H, I go back to F and maybe through to B+ as a clinching tactic.) Not only is this approach mechanical and ineffective but it also belittles the patient.

All of us are different and we shall counsel differently. What works for me may not work for you and your way of dealing with a problem may be tremendously effective when you do it, and yet seem abysmally false when I try it. So, if problem counselling cannot be learned like a set of rules, and if you already have 90% of your effectiveness within your own personality, then why bother with the 10% which remains?

Well, there is much to be gained by adding specific counselling skills into your 10%. These skills can help you to counsel more economically and more efficiently. Here are some of the counselling skills which others have found useful, and that you also may find helpful and be able to adapt for your own use.

Listening

This is an absolutely vital skill, and is covered elsewhere in this book. Sufficient for me to add just a few comments. Most people can only give full attention to another person for a short period of time. Your own mind may wander away to remembering a similar experience to the one the person is speaking about, or you may be wondering what is happening to the newly admitted patient. You may even be deciding what food to buy for the evening meal. Sometimes you will return from a personal reverie in time to hear the person saying ' . . . and I've never told that to anyone before because I feel so bad about it . . . ' and you missed it!

Practice will help you to lengthen your attention span, but even so there are times when you will need to stop the flood of disclosure with a reflecting response or a clarification question. At other times you will just need to say that you were with him/her whilst talking about . . . but missed the bit after that.

Factors which help one to listen more adequately include steady but inoffensive eye contact, attending to seating arrangements including angle, proximity and height, ability to sit quietly without interrupting, and not searching for something reassuring to say as soon as he finishes speaking. Reassurance often sounds hollow (particularly if he hasn't finished telling you the whole story) and subsequent events don't always turn out to be the bed of roses we have promised. Because the aim in problem counselling is for the person to come up with their own solutions, then we do not need to distract ourselves by puzzling out what we are going to advise. Instead we can give full attention to what the person is saying and the feelings he is expressing.

Questioning

I believe that questioning can be a nursing preoccupation, used randomly like a blunderbuss. Novice counsellors tend to ask too many questions so that the person may feel cornered, backed up against the wall, facing an inquisition. The person's need to tell his story at his own pace is sadly subverted and he may finish up by answering a barrage of questions and never get a chance to tell you what is really upsetting him. The irony of it is that the novice counsellor may go away highly pleased with having remembered to ask all the important questions and filled the interview form with facts.

Obviously there is a place for form-filling and getting the facts. My contention here is that if we are hoping to form the sort of counselling relationship in which a person feels safe to share real problems with us, then it is important not to deflect him with yet more questions, particularly when he becomes silent, speculative, looks inside himself and is obviously moving deeper into the nub of the problem. It is important not to interrupt at this stage.

Having stressed the disruptive quality of too many questions, there is of course a real place for questioning, and there are skills which can make the questions more productive.

Closed questions like 'Did you like the new timetable?' can be answered with a 'Yes' or a 'No' and do not give much information. Open questions like 'What do you think of the new timetable?' will usually lead to a longer answer and more information. Biased questions such as 'You'll have had your tea?', 'You're not going to leave him again are you?' and 'Are you wearing that for a bet?', beggar the question, expressing the answer you want to hear. Many people feel railroaded into giving you the answer you want, but then don't necessarily do what you wish them to do. 'Good morning, how are we today?' might be answered less trivially if you said 'How are you feeling this morning?'

Multiple questions pose a real problem in deciding which to answer first, and not remembering the half of them. 'How is your husband then, he's a railwayman isn't he? Does he have long to go for retirement? and what will he do then?'

Hors d'oeuvre questions

This is a concept of mine used to describe a process of trying to help a person to get in touch with his feelings, but in fact hindering him in doing so. When a hostess offers a salver of hors d'oeuvre, not many of her guests will say 'Thank you, but I don't want any of these, what I really want is . . . ' Likewise, when you as a counsellor say, 'So how are you feeling now, are you happy, apprehensive, fed up, cross?' It may well be that none of the alternatives you offer are what he wants, but he may think that he ought to pick one. Also this can be an easy option rather than having to search for the accurate description. If you simply ask 'How are you feeling right now?', you are more likely to get nearer the truth.

Reflecting

Reflecting what the person has just said to you can be unbelievably effective. There are two ways of doing this: by repeating verbatim and by paraphrasing. Reflecting verbatim helps to highlight the significance of what the person has just said. It is better used sparingly than as a maddening echo of everything the person says. It is also better to repeat only small phrases so that you can remember the words and the nuances of speech accurately. Hear-

ing a verbatim reflection of what he has just said will often lead
to the person looking more closely into that thought and those
feelings; sometimes leading to the person altering his statement
to something more accurate.

Reflecting by paraphrasing means that you use your own words
to reflect back what you have heard. If your paraphrasing is spot-
on, it can give the person a very real experience of having been
heard and understood. So then it is worth him trying to tell you
more because, somehow, you have managed to come alongside
him and have appreciated what he is feeling. If your paraphrasing
was not quite what he meant then he has a chance to rectify that,
and, once again experience the pleasure of having restated more
accurately. Don't forget also that reflecting stems a flood of information and allows you to check out that you are hearing properly.

Clarifying

This is another similar technique used to check out whether or
not what you heard is what he meant. For this you probably
have sentences of your own. Here are some sentences seeking
clarification which are known to work.

1. 'Hold on a minute, I want to check whether or not I've got this
   right. Did you say . . . ?'
2. 'Correct me if I'm wrong, what I think you are saying is . . . '
3. 'Hey, a lot of things have been happening to you. You've told
   me a lot already and I need to go a little slower so that I can
   take it in. You said . . . is that right?'
4. 'I think I understand what you said about . . . and also the
   next bit you told me about . . . but I'm not sure that I'm at all
   clear about . . . , could you tell me that again in a simpler way
   so that I can grasp it and understand more clearly what you
   are telling me?'
5. 'Are you saying . . . ?'

There are many more sentences you can make up for yourself.
If the person really is unclear and also self-conscious about that,
then it may help for you to say something like 'I don't know but
I seem to be unusually slow this morning, could you tell me that
again in a different way, nice and slowly so that I can take it in?'
Likewise, if someone is telling you about a problem and it seems
to be all words and no feeling, then you may want to say something like, 'You know, I hear what you are saying very clearly,

and yet I don't have any picture of you in this. I've no idea how you are feeling. Please tell me how you are feeling right now.' If your clients have spent a lifetime not showing their feelings then even recognizing how they feel is difficult, never mind expressing those feelings in words. Nevertheless, if you really do think that it is important for the person to be able to get in touch with his feelings despite difficulties, then you may need to give some gentle help in sorting out the feelings from the thoughts. I listen out for the word 'that'. 'I feel *that* I don't know what is going to happen to me in here,' is a thought and not a feeling. 'I feel insecure and afraid in here,' these are feelings.

It is not at all easy to differentiate between telling somebody what you are thinking and what you are feeling. However, it might help to recognize that thinking is a cerebral function occurring in the head, whilst feelings are concerned with emotions, gut reactions. Sometimes there is a marked difference between what we think in our heads, and what we feel in our gut. If we are making an important decision then it helps to be fully aware of both aspects, what we think and what we feel. For example, 'I feel *that* it will be great to have Aunt Isa come and make her permanent home with us, that will solve so many of her problems . . . but I already feel trapped and resentful of her intrusion into our home.' Decisions based on purely cognitive assessments may turn out to be quite unacceptable to our feeling selves. Sometimes, as a nurse, you will hear a patient make a clear statement about what he thinks and what he intends to do, and yet you know instinctively that his feelings are different, maybe directly opposite to his thinking solution. It can be really helpful to the patient if you gently encourage him to check out his feelings, and review his decision accordingly.

Probing

This counselling skill is best used cautiously. Many people need to be in control of what they are going to divulge, to whom, and at what rate. Thus undue haste on the part of the counsellor to probe into the painful areas might well be counter-productive. However, if the person keeps backing off, leaving major concerns hanging in the air between you, you might first try reflecting one or two key words on a rising inflection. For example, 'I think I shall have to look for a ground floor flat but I shall be lost without my neighbours.' – 'Lost?' – 'Yes, you see I don't mix with strangers but I've just got to know the couple opposite and they are good company . . . I've felt terribly lonely since my wife died . . . '

Then probing responses can include requests like 'Would you like to tell me a bit more about that, it sounds quite upsetting?' or 'I think that this whole area is quite important to you, would you like to explore it a little more with me?' or 'This topic seems to be quite distressing for you and talking about it must be quite painful. The trouble is that I'm not at all sure that it will just go away by itself. You may have to look into it more closely to get some relief, even though opening up the wound is going to hurt.'

Having reached this point you then need to make a decision about whether you have the time to listen and support him your-self, or refer him to someone else, or whether you go on to say something like 'You're carrying a heavy burden and I think you need help with that. Do you have a really good friend or a member of your family, someone you can share this with, someone whom you know you can trust?'

In other words, you don't have to do all the counselling yourself.

Referring

There will be times when you really are too rushed to counsel and other times when you feel out of your depth and wish to hand over to someone else. It may be someone else on the ward team, or you might suggest that he would like to raise these issues with community staff when he returns home. You can also remind him of other agencies dealing with specific problems like Marriage Guidance, the Family Conciliation Service (which helps parents who are separating to make the best possible plans for any children involved), councils on alcohol and other addictions, Citizen's Advice Bureau, self-help groups like Headway for those who have suffered a head injury and their caring relatives, and/or heart surgery and their relatives, Cruse, therapists offering psycho-therapy etc. Check with other members of your team who may know more appropriate agencies, and of course, check that no one else on your team was thinking of working with this particular person and his problem before you unilaterally refer him to some-one else!

Many people referred to another agency never turn up there. It helps if you ring up and find some information on the agency which allows you to speak about it more knowledgeably to the person. Your reaction when the person initially tells you something of the problem is crucial.

Let us say that it is a sexual problem and you more or less throw up your hands in horror, say you don't know anything about it, and that he should go to a sexual problems clinic. What he might think is that you were so upset by hearing about him speaking of this problem (and yet you are the most friendly person towards him) that he is certainly not going to risk another rebuff from a stranger. It may be that you have to listen and show acceptance for the person in the predicament that he is in, and only later, when the time is right say something like, 'I've been thinking about what you told me and I'd love to be able to help you with that problem. The trouble is that I am not an expert in that field and I would like you to have the best help possible. Have you ever thought of going to . . . because they seem to have the expertise I want you to have. If you decide to go ahead then I'll bring you the telephone book and you can ring up to make an appointment with them. They may come to see you in here or they may prefer to wait until you are home and then you can go to their premises.'

No doubt the way of giving the above information will need to be altered to suit the person and yourself, but I think the important factor is that you continue to show concern and non-judgemental acceptance of the person.

Confronting

Confronting is done for various reasons. For highlighting ambiguities: 'Yesterday you said such and such but today you seem to be saying something else, almost the opposite. Can you tell me what is behind this shift?' For checking intentions: 'You've said that you will do this before, but when it came to the point you didn't. What's going to be different about this time?'

If you are confronting someone, or giving them negative feedback as it is sometimes (incorrectly) termed, then it makes a whole lot of difference whether the feedback was sought or unwanted by the person. 'Tell me how you think I can improve and what I'm doing wrong,' can often lead to useful changes in behaviour. Calling someone in to your office and saying 'I'm highly dissatisfied with your performance, either you buck up your ideas or else you're out,' may lead to useful changes too, but the feelings will be different!

If you have built up a good trusting relationship with the person you are counselling then it is usually possible to confront in a reasonable manner. Even so, when you confront someone you may get emotionally charged scenes with tears, anger, counter-accusations etc.

Sometimes high feelings and raised voices spring from the patient, but at other times they arise from the nurse. Maybe it is the nurse who is angry and bitter, bringing disruption into the relationships she makes with others.

For those people who are counselling and, if anything, trying to avoid giving challenging feedback, the following format might be of some help. Remember that this is only one way and you may already have other methods of confronting which work effectively for you. Even so, you may like to try this out as an exercise with a colleague taking the role of the person you wish to confront.

1. Let the person know that you have something to say.
2. Tell him the specific behaviour you would like changed.
3. Say what effect this piece of behaviour has on you.
4. Suggest what changes you think need to be made.
5. Invite the person to comment.

These additional points will help with the above exercise.

1. Decide how long the discussion is likely to last and if the person doesn't have time right then, don't just reduce the time you need to something like a rushed two minutes. Instead, agree on a meeting when both of you do have time. When the meeting is taking place it probably helps if you are both sitting. Certainly it doesn't help to have the person hovering over you, facing the door, and making it clear that there are really far more important things to be done instead of listening to you rabbiting on about something.
2. Telling the specific behaviour you would like to see changed, not 'I'm sick of the way you always . . . ', or 'It's just like you, you're never . . . ' In other words, do not make a global disparagement including all the things that have sickened you in the last ten years. This will only put the person on the defensive and undermine the likelihood of change. If the person casts up things he doesn't like about you, or your behaviour, then you will need to ask him not to do that either. It is better to make another time to discuss other issues instead of trying to settle everything at once.

3. Saying the effect on your feelings of the specific piece of behaviour is usually the most effective part of this five-point plan for confronting. Often the person had no idea of how deeply you were affected by the specific piece of behaviour, and just hearing this is all that is necessary for change.
4. So be clear what change you would like and express it clearly.
5. Inviting the person to comment has to do with seeking agreement and commitment towards this change.

Focusing

This is a skill worth acquiring. When the person is trying to tell you as much as possible before you have to go away and do something else, it can help if you and he can decide on the bit which is most important to be focussed on and discussed in the ten minutes you have available right now. Though it is the person and not you who will be deciding on the course of action he might want to take, you can help him to focus on the different options open, and their likely effects.

Summarizing

Summarizing is a similar skill. There is a lot to be said for the person doing this instead of the counsellor and certainly, this can be revealing. Matters discussed which you thought were key points may hardly be remembered by the person. Instead his summary may tell you of things uppermost in his mind which are entirely different from your perceptions. Usually, when I am problem counselling I ask the person to jot down a few notes and produce them next time (always remembering that not everyone is able to do a task like this, not everyone is literate or physically capable of writing).

If the person does write his own notes he can produce them next time you meet. That way the person takes responsibility for his own notes and is not wondering who else is reading all about him in the office. At the next meeting it is important for the person to start with what is uppermost for him, very recent events may have overtaken the matters we have discussed last time. If not, then the summary of the previous meeting can be a good place to start; particularly as there may be additions or alterations he might wish to tell you about, and then you move on together to other topics he wishes to air.

Self disclosure

Just occasionally and not very often it may be helpful for you to reveal to a patient that you yourself have had a problem which is similar to his. Indeed it is acting upon this theory that self-help groups share their experiences so supportively. However, a few words of warning before you rush out to tell all.

The way that you solved your problem might not be the preferred solution for your client, and you may need to ensure that he doesn't adopt your solution purely because he respects you and your professional judgement.

Sometimes a person will say that you cannot possibly understand his difficulties unless you have had the same trouble as he has. I personally have worked with a lot of people with lots of different problems and I haven't found it necessary to have had a double amputation, a head injury, a stroke, an alcohol problem, blindness, multiple sclerosis etc. in order to understand when a man shares his worries and distress.

We are all of us different in the amount of personal material we are prepared to share with others, which material, and with which others. Some counsellors freely share their own thoughts, feelings and events which have happened to them. Others will not wish to share anything personal at all with the person they are counselling. Each of us needs to know where we are putting our own boundaries on this one. Certainly it could be considered unusual for a counsellor to take over the whole of a session talking about his feelings and worries, the person not getting a look in. If you are a sharer, make sure that you can trust the person first; you may not want to overhear your personal confidences being shared out of context in the day room, the health centre or the supermarket. Likewise if you let nothing of yourself through to the person he may find this extremely discomforting and clam up himself. Certainly it is important that we are genuine and not pretending to be something we are not.

Because self awareness is one of the vital qualities of a good counsellor, opportunities to share thoughts and feelings in peer groups are vital. Such training will make it easier to appreciate the difficulties experienced by persons we counsel, and make us safer practitioners.

Highlighting assets

Care is needed that we do not reduce a person's wholeness and turn him into a list of problems. The Weed system of problem-orientated records as used by some doctors, is a neat way of highlighting problems, agreed treatment measures and subsequent results. The Nursing Process documentation can provide similar information for nurses. Both of these systems can consequently reduce a person until he becomes a mere list of problems. We need to highlight a person's strengths as well as problems in order to maintain a realistic balance.

It helps to underline aspects of life which are going well. The person needs to be able to identify and use his assets because these are the strengths on which he can rebuild his life. When I have been elucidating problems I like to make a specific request, and that is that the person tells me two things which are going really well for him right now. Some persons take a long while to do this, but I just sit and wait. When it comes it may be that a favourite grandchild is doing well at school, or there are plans for the visit of an old friend, enjoying being in the garden, or whatever.

There are more skills and different approaches to counselling than I have included in this chapter, and I do hope that my short list will have given you the incentive to follow up with experiential training and reading on the subject. Note, for instance, that I have said nothing at all about the counselling of dying persons and the bereaved. I do not want to try and cram such important concepts into a few paragraphs. Instead, I wish to refer you to two books recommended in the bibliography which ends this chapter. One is *Facing Death* by Averil Stedeford and the other *Grief Counselling and Grief Therapy* by William Worden. Nor have I said anything about different styles of counselling like Transactional Analysis, person-centred counselling, the Heimler method, or the Gestalt approach which is my own favourite. Instead of trying to cover these and other styles, I would like to spend a little more time sharing with you some of the difficulties I find in the counselling process.

Don't necessarily assume that your patient will choose you to hear about his depression or family problems, or indeed any of his emotional difficulties. The person may gratefully trust you with the management of his intravenous infusion and his bladder washout etc., but this doesn't automatically mean that he will also want you to help him deal with emotional problems. He may have someone else in mind to do that, or he may be one of these people who never share worries with anyone. You may be very clear that this person's worries are the main cause of his lack of progress, but he has the right to refuse your help.

The gusher

Some people have been locked in their emotions and worries for so long that when they do find someone in whom they can confide, the story pours out, the tears flow and the anger follows. Events which have caused hurt, grief and guilt are followed by even more self-disclosure, self-loathing and pain, and the next time you see him he may avoid you like the plague, hide, discharge himself, because he has shared far too much at once and you are the most dangerous person he knows, dragging out all that information; things he had never told anyone else before! Maybe you were too active for too long with your probing. Maybe you sat tight and said absolutely nothing. Maybe you just wanted him to get maximum release of all this painful stuff so he would feel better, afraid there might not be another time like this when it would be just right.

The best thing to do with someone who gushes is to stop them. I say something like 'Oh dear, you seem to have had some awful things happening to you, one terrible thing after another. I'm getting swamped just listening, so goodness knows what it must be like for you. I find the pace of this too fast and I want to slow you down. This isn't the only time we shall have together, we can meet again tomorrow for another fifteen minutes and again after that, so we don't need to say it all now. Could you please go back to the incident you told me about when . . . and we'll try and look at that a little deeper. For example, you told me . . . that can't have been too much fun! How did you deal with it?'

Doorstep communications

Sometimes the person you are counselling tells you the most important thing when he is on the doorstep on the way out at the end of the interview. That is not by accident. He knows that you have planned to do other things now and so you won't have time to deal with it. You know that an extra five minutes is not really possible and in any case it is going to take a lot longer than five minutes to deal with this. I say, 'I think that what you have just told me is really important and unfortunately I just don't have time left to deal with it just now. Let's meet again at 2 o'clock tomorrow and I want you to be sure and start off with what you have said just now. It is important isn't it and we shouldn't try and cram this into a mere five minutes?!'

Confidentiality

If you have given assurances of absolute confidentiality and then your client says 'Well I'll see how it goes but I do have some pills if necessary,' how do you deal with that? There is no way that you can mount a 24-hour watch on a potentially suicidal person by yourself, neither can you withhold any notes you have made on a person if the courts tell you that you must present them there. So absolute confidentiality is something that we cannot offer. You may well go about things in a different way, but what I am doing these days is to say to patients, 'The things that you and I talk about will normally stay in this room, just between you and me. However, other people are concerned with your progress, your consultant, the social worker and the ward sister. If you and I discuss anything and I think other members of the staff team need to know in order to adjust your treatment in any way, I will want to tell them. After all we are a professional team and we work as a team, is that all right?' Most people say yes and we get on with it. If a person hesitates then I say, 'If I am going to share something with your doctor, then I will tell you first what I shall be telling them. Is that Okay?' I say these things on the first interview to avoid any subsequent problem of needing to inform my colleagues of something important, but having specifically or tacitly given a promise that I will not do so.

Projection

One reason why I stress the necessity of self-awareness is to encourage counsellors to discover their true strengths and use them effectively in their work. Another is to protect persons from counsellors' projections. On occasion I have looked at a person and decided that he was quite angry, or close to tears, or whatever. After I have worked with that person a little longer it has become obvious that the person is not experiencing those feelings at all: I had those feelings, and carried them into the interview from something happening in my own life. It is also possible to get into difficulties by deciding that if I had been in the situation that this person was in, I should have thought so and so and felt so and so. Therefore that person must be thinking and feeling the same as I would. This is often a false assumption, the person may be feeling and thinking something entirely different, and my projecting my feelings on to him is manifestly confusing. It really is important that we can differentiate clearly between what is us, and what is the person we are working with.

Confluence

When two rivers join and flow together it becomes practically impossible to tell which is which, they just merge into one. Sometimes you may have the experience of working with a person who is so much like yourself that you are confluent with them. It is singularly difficult to counsel a person who is almost identical with you and most counsellors will pull out because they are not effective nor objective.

Anxiety

Sometimes the anxiety level of the person is so high that normal communication is impossible. Tunnel vision, hearing only what he wants to hear or is afraid to hear, misunderstanding and fright, are uppermost. There may indeed be a physical cause for this, such as an impending heart attack, a haemorrhage, bad news etc. Having checked that and if nothing needs to be done immediately, then you might be better giving a short relaxation session and attending to the breathing, rather than trying to use other counselling skills. Find one of your colleagues who is good on relaxation skills. This may be another nurse, a physiotherapist, an occupational therapist or a psychologist. Be sure that as well as seeing how this is done, you also learn one of the relaxation methods which suits you. This is something which can be of real use for yourself as well as your patients.

And do remember to finish off the relaxation session slowly, avoiding jerky movements which may aggravate old injuries, also be sure that the person is properly alert before driving off in his car.

Staying in the here and now

Psychoanalysts and some psychotherapists spend a lot of time going back over events in early life. This takes a lot of time but can be productive. On the other hand people who are counselling, and have only a very limited time to do this, are better to deal with what is happening here and now, and to deal with present feelings too. Thus, if a person is recounting past events to you, you may wish to say something like 'You have been telling me about . . . which happened . . . ago, and I'm wondering how that is affecting you now. How are you feeling right now?' Or, 'What you have just told me is obviously important and it has certainly made an impression on you, to the point where it is still vivid in your memory to this day. Yet, to some extent, that is water under the bridge now, do you think that anything needs to be done about it now? Is there anything you can do about it now? What do you need to do in order to sort it? Is there some way in which you can finish this business and then get it out of your thoughts? It will be an awful shame if what happened so long ago is still going to affect your enjoyment of life here and now.'

Stress

To the myriad books and articles already written on nurses' stress and burnout, I would add a few brief comments of my own. There are no prizes for cracking up emotionally. It seems to be the best nurses who suffer burnout, the ones who give and give of themselves to others without thinking of their own needs. Being supportive and empathic with a person in trouble means getting involved, standing alongside, and feeling some of the person's pain. Add to that the stressful background of staff shortages, workload, lack of a quiet room and the pressures mount.

There has to be some way that nurses can deal with their own stress, and I offer a few ideas to add to your own strategies.

1. Reading about stress.
2. Learning to recognize the signs of stress in yourself.
3. Identifying precursors of stress in your home and your work environment, and actually doing something about reducing these.
4. Ensuring that your work with patients does not exclude other interests in your life – visiting friends, reading, going to concerts, films, exhibitions, sporting activities, planning holidays. learning how to relax, keeping physically fit, etc.
5. Learning how to delegate and to say NO when necessary.
6. Devising effective ways of reaching decisions.
7. Revising and maybe discarding some of your hidden rules;

injunctions which were drummed into you as a child or even in your nurse training school. For example, I must always please everyone. I must never show my feelings! I must be perfect all the time! I must always think of others first, putting their needs before mine.

Take some of your own medicine. Find someone to whom *you* can off-load. No doubt you will have witnessed the easing of strain, the flood of relief which follows a good counselling session in which a person has at last been able to talk about major worries and strong feelings.

Some nurses off-load to family, friends or work colleagues. Others seriously overload themselves and then crawl around ruminating over old hurts, having lost whatever freshness and spontaneity they ever had. Not everyone finds it easy to share. However, for those who recognize the benefits of off-loading accumulated stress, there are various possibilities available.

Without breaching confidentiality it is possible to say something like, 'I have just been brought face to face with some really sad events and that has reopened all my own sadness. I suddenly thought about my own mother, how difficult it was for her . . . my regrets that I never told her . . . (tears) etc.' Such an off-loading need not take a long time. It is like a quick repair to allow you to carry on your work, with, hopefully, a longer session to follow at a more convenient time. It is important to be able to express the feelings as well as the facts.

Co-counselling

This is an organized way of two people meeting to speak about events in their lives and to express their feelings. One person starts and the other gives full attention, then half way through there is a short pause to enable the two participants to clear their minds, then the roles are reversed. Neither of the co-counsellors needs to be expensively trained. Neither of the co-counsellors needs to think of himself as a client in that the roles of counsellee and counsellor are swopped over at half time. Some people meet their co-counsellors regularly whereas others meet only when there is a specific problem. The counsellee arranges whatever contract he wishes with the counsellor. He sets his own pace, limits the depth and intensity that he wishes to go, and remains in charge of his 'therapy'.

'Facing distress' groups
Some issues seem to be better discussed in a staff group, rather than a one-to-one discussion. Having run such staff support groups four or five times a year for seven years, I would like to share some of my findings with you. Meeting for two hours per week for six consecutive weeks seemed to be just about right for groups numbering seven to twelve people plus facilitator. There was a definite benefit in mixing a wide variety of staff, enrolled nurses, staff nurses, sisters, nursing officers, hospital-based staff plus health visitors and community nurses. Also there was one course which included two speech therapists, a physiotherapist and an occupational therapist, as well as nurses. Variety of job situation also improved the courses. There were nurses from different hospitals and from different wards within those hospitals. Thus they came with stress and distress from cancer wards, addiction units, young chronic sick, long stay wards, orthopaedic, rehabilitation, intensive care, and chest, face and throat surgery etc. The groups were specifically set up at the request of nurses wanting to improve their effectiveness in helping patients undergoing tests and subsequent surgery for cancer, and also for dying patients and their grieving relatives, and dealing with their own distress too. The content of these 'facing distress' groups is of course confidential to their participants, but some of the general issues can be indicated. These include the effect of stress on communication, facilitating the sharing of distress, non-verbal communication, different views on touching others, ethical aspects of humouring demented people, rational thoughts versus irrational feelings etc.

Terminal illness led to discussion on the dying and the bereaved, giving a poor prognosis, helping patients, relatives and ourselves to cope with distress, procedures associated with death in a hospital ward, death of a young child, death of a young parent preparing to leave behind a young child, own personal feelings about death, personal preferences in management of final stages, the bereavement process, unresolved grief reaction etc.

Relationships with others at work, interpersonal relationships
Dealing with anger, both other people's and our own; hostility; disinhibited and noisy behaviour; self-damaging behaviour; suicide; or working with sad, withdrawn, anxious and depressed people; supporting people who have a drastically changed body

image, mourning for lost abilities, self-blame, sexual problems accompanying disability etc. It will, of course, come as no surprise to nurses to hear that some of the worst stress came in working with inept, infuriating colleagues, up, down and across the hierarchy.

Sometimes 'facing distress' meant working in wards where the staff were not getting on with each other, to a point where the situation became quite dangerous. Contrast this with a ward where all the staff are valued, where you and your colleagues support each other when under stress. As nurses we have prime responsibility for creating the right sort of atmosphere for patients, their relatives, and all who work together there. This is a challenge and a privilege for the nurses on day duty and night duty, and if we get it right then we can all thrive.

Your power as a nurse

As a nurse you are important to sick people and are invested with real power. You are in charge of the ward, your professional role and your ability command respect, you also have the ear of the consultant and other important members of the ward team. Many people will also attribute superhuman power to you, like for example, the ability to make things better, to bring an errant member of the family into line, to know whether the person should buy a new house or prepare for an early demise.

Despite all this power, both real and unreal, there will be times when you fail to meet emotional needs, and you will feel bad about that. There may even be times when you try to avoid talking to a person because he upsets you so much and you feel that you have nothing to give. There will be times when you are counselling someone whose lifestyle, personality, morals, goals or sexual preferences are so vastly different to yours, that you find it difficult to work with him non-judgementally, vital as this is. At the same time as you are giving each person the right to be himself and make his own decisions, you do need to be clear about your own standards and maintain your own integrity.

To end this chapter, I have included my list of the qualities of a good counsellor to add to yours. There are omissions which I would like to rectify, and qualifications which I would like to add, but having given myself the same limitation of twenty minutes only, I have just let the list stand as it is.

Table 6.1 Qualities of a good counsellor

Good listener	Has resources, or knows where resources are available
Non-judgemental	
Warm	Will refer if and when appropriate
Approachable	Has a comfortable office and privacy
Genuine	No telephone or other interruptions
Mature	Looks after plants properly (so may hopefully be nourishing and supportive to clients
Confidential	
Objective	
Sense of humour	Long experience as a good counsellor
Has/makes time	Dresses appropriately
Common sense	Not easily embarrassed
Creative	Free, or fees not too expensive
Imaginative	Cares about clients
Perceptive	Has 'good vibes'
Notices non-verbals	Looks healthy
Notices what is left out	Does not use jargon, or at least translates jargon
Notices where pain is	
Focuses	Looks interested, alive and friendly
Good pacing/timing	Strong-minded and able to speak about upsetting things
Confronts appropriately	
Calm	Does not want to take over or make you like himself
Keeps fairly still	
Empathic	Encourages independence of himself and others
Knowledgeable	
Supportive	Can deal with panic, knows about physiology of anxiety, tension, stress, headaches, breathing etc.
Does not advise	
Does not preach	
Makes good, pleasing eye contact	Can recognize and deal with neurotic and psychotic behaviour

Further reading

Dryden, W. (1988) *Counselling in Action*, Sage Publications, London.

Grigor, J.C. (1986) *Loss – an invitation to grow*, Arthur James Ltd., London.

Munro, E., Mathei, R. and Small, J. (1983) *Counselling: A Skills Approach*, (Revised edition) Methuen, Bristol.

Nelson-Jones, R. (1988) *Practical Counselling Skills*, (Second edition) Holt Rinehart and Winston, London.

Stedeford, A. (1985) *Facing Death*, Heinemann, London.

Tschudin, V. (1987) *Counselling Skills for Nurses*, (Revised edition) Baillière Tindall, London.

Worden, J.W. (1982) *Grief Counselling and Grief Therapy*, Tavistock, London.

7

Discipline

Nancy MacLeod Nicol

7.1. What is discipline?

Discipline is something with which you are all familiar. However, it is amazingly difficult to answer questions such as 'What is discipline?' or 'What purpose does it serve?' Most of you have had experience of being responsible for discipline – perhaps as a school prefect, a Patrol Leader in Guides or Scouts, or in a previous job and also, on the receiving end, of chastisement by parents, teachers or charge nurses.

The word discipline has many different meanings. The first meaning denotes a mode of life in accordance with rules. Many of you play games, whether they are physically active like hockey, badminton or curling or more passive such as Trivial Pursuit, Scrabble or card games. In order that you can play these games effectively you must know the rules. Mary Poppins, in the musical of that name, says 'Snap, the job's a game,' so in order to work you must know the rules.

People in our society who are responsible for maintaining discipline do not often receive thanks for carrying out what is often a hard task. Think for a moment about your views on the police, traffic wardens, teachers or nurse managers. Are they all pleasant thoughts? In your role as a staff nurse you have a responsibility to maintain discipline and many find this difficult, as no one likes to be seen as the 'baddy'. Rules make a code or discipline, and they make clear what is acceptable behaviour. Rules promote standards and have been with us for many years.

Still thinking about discipline, think of self-discipline. Parents try to teach, by example, the manners, honesty and behaviour that are expected of you by society. As time goes by you learn self-discipline when you become aware that you are responsible for your actions, getting to a stated place on time; keeping your room tidy; living within your budget, in· fact having control of yourself and your behaviour. As a staff nurse, you are a role model, teaching by example, and self-discipline is reflected, for example, by hand-washing before and after carrying out a procedure in the clinical areas, thus assisting in the control of infection. Discipline can also mean a branch of learning. You are in the nursing discipline where a professional attitude to your work means following and understanding the procedures and rules laid down by the profession.

Another meaning of discipline is to control or to correct. As a staff nurse you will be aware that your employing authority has a written *Disciplinary Policy and Procedure* which 'comes into action' when a member of staff breaks the rules or policies. Then the 'offender' is corrected. Just as parents and mentors throughout life guide you to control yourself, they equally exercise control in guiding you to the correct approach, in which, if you fail, you may be corrected.

Having discussed the various meanings of discipline, the next step is to think about the various laws, rules and policies which affect you as a trained nurse.

7.2. Discipline that relates to you and your work

The country in which we live has laws, Acts of Parliament and Codes of Practice which affect us both as citizens and as trained nurses. Laws which apply to us as residents of the country include those pertaining to murder, theft, fraud and drunk driving. The laws in particular which affect us as trained nurses are the care and storage of drugs, health and safety, and employment legislation.

Your employing authority has certain policies and procedures to which you are expected to adhere during your working hours. Many are made to facilitate the effective and efficient working practices of the hospital or clinic, others will provide guidance on the wearing of correct uniform, which day of the week orders are submitted, and the procedure for booking annual leave. But mainly they are concerned with disciplinary matters such as the procedures to follow when staff fail to obey the set procedures and codes of practice. Health Authority/Boards' rules may vary in different areas of the country. You should ensure that you are familiar with the rules for your own area.

As a staff nurse you have a dual responsibility, that of ensuring that your own work complies with the standards laid down by your employing authority *and* to ensure that other staff working with you appreciate these standards and the consequence of breaking them – ignorance is not innocence or an excuse!

In addition to local policies and rules of your employers every nurse is, by statute, accountable for her actions to the United Kingdom Central Council which has laid down a *Code of Professional Conduct*. A breach of this could result in the removal of the offending nurse's name from the professional register. This code whilst not being law in the usual sense is nevertheless binding. Contravention carries similar penalties to offences under the law of the land, such as theft.

The UKCC has also produced advisory documents to supplement the original code. These are as follows.

1. Exercising Accountability (1989)
2. Advertising by Registered Nurses, Midwives and Health Visitors (1985)
3. Administration of Medicines (1986)
4. Confidentiality (1987).

Professional staff at the UKCC are always willing to give advice to any nurses on matters relating to professional practice.

7.3. What is misconduct?

Although it is not an easy part of the trained nurse's function, it is necessary, on occasions, to provide guidance and to deal with matters of misconduct. Breaking the laws of the land, breaking Health Authority/Boards' policies, or failing to adhere to the Code of Professional Conduct can all be termed misconduct.

On appointment to your present position, you signed a contract of service which stated that you had read and understood the Health Authority/Board's Disciplinary Policy and Procedure. You may have been given a copy or advised where you could have access to this information. *Disciplinary Policy and Procedure* usually outlines examples of what would be considered as minor or less serious misconduct by staff (absenteeism, misuse of health service property, verbal abuse or poor workmanship). These will require counselling or warnings to ensure that they are not repeated, while examples of serious or gross misconduct (assault, theft and fraud) may result in the nurse being dismissed from her present employment.

When your name was recorded on the register with the United Kingdom Central Council you were issued with a copy of the *Code of Professional Conduct*, which states 'Each registered nurse, midwife and health visitor shall act, at all times, in such a manner as to justify public trust and confidence, to uphold and enhance the good standing and reputation of the profession, to serve the interests of society, and above all to safeguard the interests of individual patients and clients.' It states that every trained nurse is accountable for her practice and lists several clauses for guidance and advice.

However, if summary dismissal for assault on a patient occurred then the UKCC may be informed and they could remove the nurse's name from the register as the following clauses of the Code of Professional Conduct would have been breached.

Act always in such a way as to promote and safeguard the well being and interests of patients/clients.

Ensure that no action or omission on his/her part or within his/her sphere of influence is detrimental to the condition or safety of patients/clients.

Should a nurse's name be removed from the register she is not eligible for employment as a registered nurse.

As a trained nurse you must be prepared to voice your own feelings on any matter which you feel is having an adverse effect on the patient(s). You are the patients' advocate. An example where advocacy is needed may be that (because of 'various circumstances') there are not enough nurses on duty at a particular time to give satisfactory standard of patient care, or that particular resources are not available, for example, bed linen, pyjama trousers. Such matters must be brought to the attention of your senior nurse and follow it up in writing and collect any evidence pertinent to the case. Lack of time and red tape should not mean that you ignore your professional responsibilities. You are a professional nurse with professional accountability to 'have regard to the environment of care and its physical, psychological and social effects on patients/clients, and also to the adequacy of resources, and make known to appropriate persons or authorities any circumstances which could place patients/clients in jeopardy or which militate against safe standards of practice.' You are also expected to 'have regard to the workload of and the pressures on professional colleagues and subordinates, and take appropriate action if these

Figure 7.1 A Statement of Competence

STATEMENT OF COMPETENCE

ADDITION OF DRUGS TO INTRAVENOUS INFUSIONS

Surname .... Forenames................................

Grade .... PIN ....

This is to certify that the above named person has successfully completed a programme of theoretical and practical instruction in the said procedure and is prepared to introduce drugs into (1) Bottles/Bags (2) burette.

Instructor/s signature and grade

1)... 2)..
Date ....

Assessor/s signature and grade

1)...2)..
Date ....

Director of Nursing Services signature ....
Date ....

Administrative Consultant signature...
Date ....

I...
am willing to assume responsibility as required in accordance with the LHB Extended Clinical Role of the Nurse Policy.

Date ....

The holder of a statement of competence is authorised to carry out the above procedure in accordance with the Lothian Health Board and Royal Infirmary of Edinburgh 'Extended Clinical Role of The Nurse Policy' having satisfied her/himself that she/he feels competent to do so and is willing to accept the responsibility delegated to her/him.

are seen to be such as to constitute abuse of the individual practitioner and/or to jeopardize safe standards of practice.'

You must also be aware of the workload of the members of the staff. It is all too easy for one unfortunate learner to receive orders and instructions from every member of the ward team as she is the only nurse in sight! Or, that as the nurse in charge you fail to inform your nurse manager that someone is not on duty (perhaps because she had overslept).

This can cause anxiety, stress and affects safe practice of patient care.

At all times you must ensure the best for your patients.

The extended role of the nurse is not a new role; but it can mean carrying out procedures which, in the past, have often been undertaken by the medical staff. At present, a qualified nurse is trained in the procedure by the medical staff or charge nurse. Having demonstrated her competence satisfactorily, a document is completed according to the Health Authority/Board's policy.

The extended role is not transferable, further training is required when a nurse transfers to another ward, department or hospital. This is for reasons of legality rather than competence. It is stressed that you do not undertake, or delegate to others, tasks or procedures in which you or they have not been trained. Most learners readily tell you what they have not been taught in the classroom, but beware, some do not. They may want the glamour or excitement of doing something different.

Therefore you have a responsibility to be knowledgeable about what is taught and when, during a student or pupil nurse's training. If you fail to do this you have placed yourself in a position where you are liable to be subject to action from the United Kingdom Central Council, having contravened the clause which states, 'Acknowledge any limitations of competence and refuse in such cases to accept delegated functions without first having received instruction in regard to those functions and having been assessed as competent.'

However, in reality everything is not so simple that all misconduct is set out as black or white. There are many grey areas where misconduct could have happened for a variety of reasons. The nurse may not have carried out a procedure according to Health Authority/Board's policy or it may have been that the correct equipment to carry out that procedure was not available; or perhaps the nurse was asked to perform a procedure for which she had no instruction or training.

A thorough investigation of any misconduct must be made, and it is therefore essential that all relevant facts are at hand and that the 'offending' nurse has had the opportunity to give her side of the situation, especially in circumstances where further action could involve the implementation of the disciplinary procedure.

7.4. Professional guidance

Some Health Authorities/Boards wrongly use the word counselling as a precursor to disciplinary action, however, guidance and advice are considered by others to be more acceptable words. Guidance should form part of the action programme with any nurse who is a poor performer. This guidance is not part of the disciplinary procedure, but advice must have been given before the procedure can be implemented.

Often nurses say that they have not been advised regarding their performance, however, on closer questioning they agree that they had been 'spoken to' or 'had a talk about' the offence. The guidance in this context involves several stages.

1. Discussion on performance standards.
2. Agreement that there has been a breach of standards.
3. Confirmation of responsibility for this fault.
4. Confirmation of method of correction.
5. Agreement on a date for reviewing the action taken.

Nurse managers recognize that giving constructive advice to staff is an ongoing procedure which will help to ensure that policies and standards are being upheld. The manager informs the nurse that she has not upheld the policy laid down and indicates the action (or non-action) by the nurse which has led to this breach of conduct, and clearly indicates the behaviour expected from the nurse in the future. In cases where guidance is either not appropriate (gross misconduct) or it is not having the desired effect, it will be necessary to take formal disciplinary action.

When would you advise a nurse, and who takes action? Here is an example.

A staff nurse seldom comes on duty on time, and in fact in the past two days she has been twenty minutes late in reporting on duty each day. She is confronted by the charge nurse when she

admits that she knows she is late, but says she will make up the
time at the end of the shift. The charge nurse points out that
making up time is not the issue, coming on late puts an extra
burden on the other nurses. The charge nurse can then ask for an
explanation for her lateness. It may be that she suffered morning
sickness, or a relative at home was ill. If that is the case then help
should be offered. However, if the reason is oversleeping and/or
missing transport, then the charge nurse advises the staff nurse
that unless her time keeping improves within a week, it will be
necessary to implement the first stage of the disciplinary procedure
by issuing an oral warning after the week has elapsed if no
improvement is noted.

7.5. Disciplinary policy

Where procedures have been laid down and any misconduct has
occurred, disciplinary action may be used to prevent the recur-
rence of the situation. Any disciplinary policy which does not have
this type of correction as its objective is valueless. With the present
high cost of recruitment, both in time and money, and the difficulties in the National Health Service of obtaining and retaining
staff, the importance of effective corrective action for misconduct
has real meaning.

The emphasis of any disciplinary policy should be on correction
rather than punishment, with sufficient time for the nurse in
question to improve her performance.

7.5.1. Disciplinary procedure

A recognized disciplinary procedure is necessary if staff are to be
treated in a consistently fair manner in cases of alleged failure to
meet the standard of conduct laid down by the employing authority. It should be stressed that this procedure is intended to be used
to correct and improve standards of behaviour and performance, it
is not a means of administering punishment.

Many nurses take the attitude that disciplinary action is something that happens, but does not affect them, until it does!
Assumptions are made by managers that staff should know better.
Too often local rules and standards of conduct are inadequately
defined, poorly communicated or written in legal jargon. It is the
responsibility of the employer to set standards and communicate

them to the staff in language that they can understand, stipulating what is required of them.

It is very important that the procedure is correctly followed. It can be difficult for the inexperienced manager to view a situation objectively, and it is advisable that guidance is sought from the immediate superior and the Personnel Officer before any action is taken, as whenever there is a policy and procedure there is a need for people who are skilled in interpreting it in relation to a particular situation. This skill can be acquired with greater understanding of the rules and with experience.

So adequate preparation is necessary before commencing the disciplinary procedure. In conducting the disciplinary interview the manager brings together knowledge and skills in order to act fairly, both to the employing authority and to the nurse concerned. Often the outcome of disciplinary action depends on how well, or how badly this interview has been conducted.

7.5.2. Following the procedure

Oral warning

An oral warning is the first stage of the disciplinary procedure relating to minor offences or unsatisfactory conduct. It is normally used when guidance previously given in counselling is not heeded by the nurse concerned. In certain circumstances it may be appropriate to give an oral warning without prior counselling. An example of this is when a nurse clearly knew, without having to be told, that what she was doing was unacceptable and what the consequences would be. For example, abusive language.

Despite the terminology, an oral warning should be recorded in the nurse's personal file and retained there for the right period. In some circumstances, it may be beneficial to follow up the oral warning by a letter to her setting out the improvement required, confirming any training etc. offered by management and advising her of her right to appeal.

Prior to an oral warning being issued the following 'basic principles' must be followed.

1. Make a proper investigation to obtain the facts.
2. Give the nurse the opportunity to explain herself.
3. Be objective and rational.
4. Follow the correct procedure.

(a) Give the nurse time to consult her Trade Union or Staff Representative.
(b) Take into account related offences.
(c) Ensure the nurse knows of her right to appeal.

The aim of this stage of the disciplinary procedure is that the nurse has a chance to improve.

First written warning

This is the second stage of the disciplinary procedure, usually implemented when a nurse has disregarded an oral warning (which is still valid, that is, within the agreed period) and has not improved her conduct or performance. It may, however, on occasions, be appropriate to issue a first written warning as the first stage of the procedure, given the relative seriousness of the misconduct or poor performance. If this action is taken, advice should be sought from the Personnel Officer. Prior to issuing such a warning, ensure that the basic principles noted under 'oral warning' have been followed, and that the nurse is aware that failure to improve may lead to the next stage of the disciplinary procedure, that of a final warning. A first written warning is retained on a nurse's personal file for a period in accordance with local agreement.

Final written warning

This stage of the disciplinary procedure follows the first written warning when a nurse has repeated the misconduct or has not made any improvement in her performance during the period when the first written warning was still valid. Prior to issuing such a warning, again the basic principles noted under 'oral warning' are followed. The nurse is advised that failure to improve may lead to the next stage of the disciplinary procedure which is dismissal.

First and final warning

This type of warning is issued when an offence is committed which is sufficiently serious that earlier stages of the procedure would not be appropriate, and dismissal would be too harsh a decision. The nurse would be given the opportunity to improve her performance whilst being informed that a single repetition of the same or related misconduct would most likely lead to her dismissal. As with previous warnings the basic principles noted under 'oral warning' would be followed.

Dismissal

The final stage of the procedure is the termination of the nurse's contract of employment – dismissal. There are two types of dismissal.

1. Dismissal following a final warning or a first and final warning disciplinary procedure.
2. In a case of gross misconduct a decision to dismiss can be taken without going through the warning stages of the procedure. This type of dismissal is called summary dismissal. Gross misconduct constitutes a breach of contract and as such the manager is not obliged to offer any period of notice or payment in lieu of notice. Again the basic principles of the procedure would be followed prior to issuing a dismissal.

7.6. Understanding the procedure

For many the policy and procedure is obscured by the phraseology used, and a lawyer rather than a dictionary may be required to understand what is meant. Several Health Authorities/Boards' *Disciplinary Policy and Procedure* are accompanied by explanatory notes which cover the following topics.

Collecting information

It is important to seek out facts and distinguish them from opinions, gossip, guesses and assumptions however minor the incident, before any disciplinary action is considered. When statements of witnesses are required these should be provided by the individuals and signed.

Correspondence and records

It is very important that records are kept of all disciplinary actions. Nurses who are given written warnings or who are dismissed must have the decision and reason for the decision confirmed in writing, and be told how they can appeal against them. Letters regarding disciplinary matters are normally sent by recorded delivery. Copies of correspondence will be kept in the nurse's personal file and copies sent to the Personnel Officer. Any relevant documentation such as statements from witnesses, or accident/incident forms should also be filed. The offending nurse's Trade Union or Staff Association have a right to see this information to assist them when they act as her representative.

Nature of complaint

The nurse must be informed of the complaint against her and be given every opportunity to state her case before any decision is taken. One offence must not be used for punishing her for other unsatisfactory behaviour. For example, a nurse who comes on duty late should not have that reason used when considering a further offence involving procedure or poor workmanship.

Extension of an existing warning

There can be circumstances where progression to the next stage of the disciplinary procedure is considered too harsh, but some form of action is essential. This situation most frequently occurs when a nurse is on a 'final' or 'first and final' warning, and who commits another misdemeanour which requires action, but where dismissal is considered inappropriate despite the previous record. The manager may, in consultation with the Personnel Officer, re-affirm the existing warning, for example in the case of a 'final warning' or 'first and final warning', to extend the period of warning by a further year.

Other circumstances

Evidence often includes other circumstances. The age of a nurse may be important – a young person 'who may be led astray' – older people 'who should have known better' or a nurse nearing retirement. Long and previous good service may well affect the decision taken.

Representation

Nurses need a voice that will be heard and heeded, a collective voice. This voice is known as a Trade Union or Professional Organization. Every nurse has a right to belong to a union, and in fact should be encouraged to do so. Nurses may belong to professional organizations, for example the Royal College of Nursing and Royal College of Midwives, where all members will be of the same profession. She may wish to join a Trade Union where other members are doing the same or similar work, for example the

Confederation of Health Service Employees (COHSE), the National and Local Government Officers' Association (NALGO) or the National Union of Public Employees (NUPE).

1. The nurse being interviewed regarding an alleged offence which may lead to discipline must be informed of her right to be accompanied by a representative of her Trade Union or Staff Association, or by a friend or colleague. Reasonable time must be allowed for the nurse to obtain representation.

2. When a Shop Steward or Staff Representative is the subject of the investigation which could lead to disciplinary action she is entitled to be represented from the outset by the full-time official or other senior lay representative designated by the union for that purpose and, therefore, before proceeding with the investigation the Manager should contact the Personnel Officer who will advise the Union or Staff Association accordingly. The reason for this action is to protect management from accusations of victimization of a Shop Steward and to avoid any misunderstandings on either side about how the Shop Steward exercises his Trade Union duties.

   (All nurses have the right to participate in union activities outside working hours, but not to have time off during working hours for union activities or for industrial action unless an agreement has been made with management. Shop Stewards are allowed more flexibility but activities within working hours should take place at a time mutually convenient with management.)

Right of appeal

When a nurse considers that the disciplinary decision taken against her is unfair, she may appeal to a higher level of management not previously involved. The nurse must be advised to whom (depending on the policy of the area) she can appeal and that she should do so within twenty-one days of receipt of the letter confirming the disciplinary action taken. If, for example, a first written warning was issued to a staff nurse by a sister or charge nurse, then the staff nurse may appeal to the senior nurse of the unit. In the case of an appeal against dismissal the nurse may, if she gets no satisfaction from her employing authority, take this to an Industrial Tribunal, however this only applies if she has been in employment for over two years.

Suspension

Suspension is not part of the disciplinary procedure. It should only be used to allow for an investigation to take place, as suspension can take tension out of a situation, for the sake of the nurse as well as management and other members of the staff. Suspension should be confirmed in writing, and should define the following aspects.

1. The reason for suspension.
2. The date and time from which it will operate.
3. The date on which further discussion on the incident will be considered.
4. The nurse's right to consult her Trade Union or Staff Association.

Suspension is on full pay and should not be of an unduly long period, except in exceptional circumstances.

The same or related conduct

It is not possible to give a precise definition of what constitutes 'related conduct'. Poor timekeeping and failure to report in sick are clearly related, whereas poor timekeeping and poor workmanship might not be. Each situation would have to be considered in the light of its own circumstances, and an overall view taken of the nurse's approach and attitude to her work and responsibilities.

7.7. Principles of implementation

Whilst the policy for discipline and appeals is laid down by the Area Health Authority/Board, the implementation of the policy and development of procedures will be determined by senior management. This is because the organizational structures within an area may differ and what is appropriate for one district or unit may not be so for another. Thus local application will vary. However, essential principles and standards of fairness should be maintained throughout the National Health Service. This is based on a system of clearly defined levels of authority and responsibility as indicated on Fig. 7.2.

Despite there being a set Disciplinary Policy and Procedure, there are no hard and fast rules for every 'offence' which occurs. Each case is treated on its own merits. That is why many nurses find it difficult to understand the procedure. However, as a guide

Fig. 7.3. gives examples of the various stages of the Disciplinary Procedure which may be undertaken.

Figure 7.2 Points to consider before initiating disciplinary procedure

Stage	Initiated by	Notification to	Action by	Appeal to
Oral Warning	A	B	A	B/C
First Warning	A	B	A	B/C
Final Warning	A/B	PO	B	C
First and Final Warning	A/B	PO	B	C
Dismissal	A/B	PO	C	Area

A Direct Supervision (for a staff nurse this would be the sister/charge nurse).
B Head of Department (senior nurse or nursing officer).
C The Manager with specifically delegated powers of dismissal.
PO The Personnel Officer.

Figure 7.3 Stages of Disciplinary Procedure

Persistent lateness	Unauthorized absence from place of work, but with previous good performance at work	Assault on a patient
Oral warning First written warning Final warning Dismissal	First and final warning Dismissal	Summary dismissal

7.8 Conclusion

The main aim of discipline is to improve performance. It is a formalized system used to warn a nurse that her performance or conduct within the work situation is not satisfactory and that unless she does something about it, disciplinary action will be taken.

The disciplinary procedure is laid down in accordance with the Employment Protection (Consolidation) Act (1978) and in accordance with the Advisory Conciliation and Arbitration Service Code of Practice on Disciplinary Procedures, and should allow for consistency, objectivity and impartiality in dealing with breaches of conduct.

The most common reason for disciplinary action being overturned at Appeal level is because management failed to follow the basic principles.

1. They failed to obtain sufficient information before putting the disciplinary process into action.
2. When they did, they failed to carry out the procedure correctly.

In your new management role as a staff nurse you have a responsibility to gain knowledge of your Health Authority/Board's *Disciplinary Policy and Procedure* so that you are aware of the standards of performance and behaviour expected of you, and of the staff that you supervise.

In conclusion, many staff nurses ask for real examples to gain a fuller insight into the *Disciplinary Policy and Procedure*. Here are two, each of which illustrates important areas of discipline.

It is important that all relevant information is available before you think of implementing any disciplinary action.

7.8.1. The problem of Terry Hart

Terry Hart qualified as a registered general nurse two months ago, and since then has worked as a staff nurse in a 28-bedded male medical ward. Over the past month there has been a national influenza epidemic and this has caused an increase in the number of admissions to the ward and a resultant decrease in the staffing due to sickness.

On the late shift yesterday Terry was in charge and two student nurses were also on duty. During the night one of the patients, Ian Struthers (aged thirty-two years) staggered and fell on his way to the toilet. On investigation it was discovered that Ian, a newly diagnosed diabetic, had not received his evening dose of insulin which had been prescribed earlier in the evening by the house officer.

Consider the points in Table 7.1 and the circumstances in Table 7.2.

Table 7.1 Points to consider before initiating disciplinary procedure

What circumstances would/might need to be considered before taking action?
Is this a matter of Discipline and if not, why not?
What would be appropriate action and who would take that action?

Table 7.2 Approach to the problem of Terry Hart

1. Circumstances to be considered.

(a) Was he aware of the drug policy? ....YES/NO
(b) Was the insulin prescribed before the medicine
   round was done?...YES/NO
(c) Had he received 'induction' in his role as staff
   nurse?...YES/NO

(d) Was he considered an experienced staff nurse to
   be in charge of the ward?.............................YES/NO

2. This will depend on the circumstances considered, if the answer
   to all of them is NO, then this does NOT constitute a matter
   of discipline.
   Management are at fault by not having helped Terry in his new
role.
   If the answer to all of them is YES, then this does constitute a
matter of discipline.

3. Action in the first case: professional guidance by the charge
   nurse.
   Action in the second case: oral warning by the nursing officer.

This example was used to illustrate that it is very important to
consider the circumstances as they can affect the outcome very
strongly.

7.8.2. The dilemma of Lesley Boyd

As a newly qualified staff nurse you need to be aware of your
responsibility to your professional body, the United Kingdom Central Council, for your accountability in your professional practice.
You could, on occasions, find yourself faced with a dilemma such
as this one.

Lesley Boyd, a newly qualified staff nurse, is working on a long-
stay psychiatric ward. Amongst the other nurses on the ward is
Noel Gillsland, a mature enrolled nurse, who has worked there
for several years. Lesley has become increasingly concerned whilst
on duty with Noel since she considers that Noel is 'rough-handling' patients. This behaviour is never apparent when Noel and
Lesley are on duty with the charge nurse. Noel and the charge

nurse always seem friendly. Lesley has a dilemma: can she allow the behaviour she witnesses to continue, and to whom should she go for help?

Consider the points in Table 7.3 then read Table 7.4.

Table 7.3   The young nurse's dilemma

What action should she take?
What further information is required and from whom will it be obtained?
What clause in the Code of Professional Conduct is being abused?

Table 7.4   Answers to questions posed in the nurse's dilemma

1. What action should she take?

   Discuss the problem with the charge nurse who should speak with Noel Gillsland. However, if no action is taken, Lesley should report the problem to her nursing officer.

2. What further information is required and from whom should it be obtained?

   Statements taken from any witnesses to the 'rough-handling', which could be other members of staff or patients.
   Whether the 'rough-handling' is proven or not the enrolled nurse must be made aware of the complaint against him.

3. Which clause of the Code of Professional Conduct is being breached?

   'Ensure that no action or omission on his/her part or within his/her sphere of influence is detrimental to the condition of safety of patients/clients.'

References

ACAS (1978) *Code of Practice 1 Disciplinary Practice and Procedure in Employment*, HMSO, London.

Baly, M. (1984) *Professional Accountability*, John Wiley and Sons, Chichester.

Pyne, R. (1981) *Professional Discipline in Nursing*, Blackwell Scientific Publications, Oxford.

Sykes, M. (1985) *Licensed to Practise*, Baillière Tindall, London.

United Kingdom Central Council (1984) *Code of Professional Conduct for the Nurse, Midwife and Health Visitor*, UKCC, London.

United Kingdom Central Council (1987) *Confidentiality* (Advisory Paper), UKCC, London.

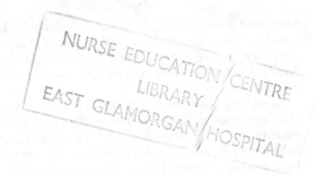

8

Moral and legal aspects of patient care

Nicola Downing

8.1. Introduction

Moral and legal issues relate to standards of behaviour in society, based on the values, attitudes and beliefs of that society (Skerry, 1983). It is important that a staff nurse understands the moral and legal aspects of her work because she is accountable for all of her actions.

Moral and legal issues are set down into codes of conduct. The legal code is decided, documented and enforced by well-established social processes, and its intention is to regulate behaviour between individuals or interest groups in society. The legal process is intended to give objective judgements of behaviour between individuals; a nurse must know the behaviour that is required of her by law. Moral codes may also be described and documented, but do not necessarily bind all members of society and cannot always be enforced (except when they overlap with the concerns of the legal code). A moral code is less definitive and less binding than a legal code, leaving more interpretation to the individual, particularly as it applies to specific issues. There are sections of society which concur in upholding certain standards of behaviour and will therefore choose to adhere to a particular moral code, for example, organized religions and the professions, whose members agree on the standards of behaviour that they expect to meet.

Behaviour is influenced by attitudes, values and beliefs. These three are closely linked, and all describe what matters to people. What people decide to be right or wrong, good or bad ultimately depends on what they consider to be important (what they value). The value placed on an object or an action depends on beliefs about that object or action, and this will be shown in the attitudes adopted toward that object or action. For example, a fur coat, a Rembrandt painting and helping an old lady across the road may or may not be perceived as valuable depending on beliefs held about them, and attitudes toward them will vary individually.

It may or may not be believed that it is exploiting animals to kill them for the adornment of the human race, that it enhances civilization to encourage the pursuit of excellence embodied in the decorative arts and that society should protect its weaker members. The value placed on the coat, the painting and the deed will depend on which of the relevant beliefs are held. The attitude exhibited toward an old lady in a mink coat buying a Rembrandt will depend on these beliefs and values.

The obvious scope for disagreement between individuals about particular beliefs illustrates the difficulties faced by society in formulating moral codes, i.e., in deciding what is right and wrong, and shows why moral codes cannot be definitive or enforceable. But although moral codes cannot incorporate all the views of all individuals, there is in fact, a large element of agreement within society concerning fundamentally important beliefs. Fundamental issues on which any moral code is based include beliefs about the meaning and purpose of human life, beliefs about the place of mankind in the world, about the forces which guide the universe and have powers of creation. In other words beliefs about life and death. Membership of a profession implies acceptance of the values, beliefs and attitudes (the moral code) of that profession (Schrock, 1990).

In the United Kingdom, the United Kingdom Central Council is the organizing body of the nursing profession, and when it was formed in 1983 following the Nurses' Act of 1979, it was stated that its principal function is to 'establish and improve standards of training and professional conduct' (Pyne 1988).

In order to fulfil this function the UKCC produced a *Code of Professional Conduct* to guide the behaviour of nurses (UKCC 1984). This guidance must be agreed by the practising nurses who make up the profession, and it is therefore important that nurses examine the issues which the Code of Conduct addresses.

Examining the moral issues which concern nursing practice means embarking on a study of ethics. Morals describe right and wrong – the principles of what is considered to be good or evil. Ethics is the study of the practice of moral behaviour, i.e., what one ought to do. The study of ethics involves a systematic investi-

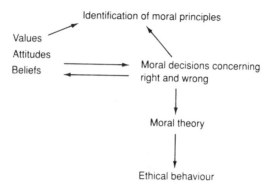

Figure 8.1 Derivation of ethical behaviour from moral principles

gation of what influences behaviour; it means identifying values, attitudes and beliefs and clarifying how they are embodied in moral principles. Briefly, the steps in this organization can be understood according to Fig. 8.1.

The capacity to understand and interpret moral codes is important in view of the fact that society is in a constant state of change and moral decisions have to incorporate change. Just as the values of an individual change, adapt and broaden with increased experience of life and exposure to new situations, so the values of society change to meet contemporary needs. For example in twentieth-century British society, scientific advances giving greater control over health and awareness of environmental damage threatening the continuation of life on Earth have both influenced values and beliefs of individuals which are reflected in the standards of behaviour which they adopt (i.e., they choose their moral codes). Nurses in the UK are asked to accept the Code of Professional Conduct (the moral code) of the UKCC; when they do this they agree to comply with standards of behaviour based on the beliefs and values of a caring profession in a Christian society. The main statements introducing the UKCC Code identify the following principles.

1. Professional accountability.
2. The primacy of the interest of the individual patient/client.

In accepting these principles a nurse must understand how they will apply in practice.

8.2. Professional accountability

Implicit in the status of a profession is the acceptance of account-ability for actions. This acceptance assumes that the actions of a professional are firmly based on appropriate knowledge, under-standing and expertise (Hull, 1980 pp. 702–12).

The UKCC has clearly stated that nurses accept professional accountability; the nurse is accountable to the public, to her pati-ent/client, to her employer and to her profession. The UKCC details the ways that accountability is exercised in nursing practice (UKCC 1989); underlying them is an assumption of an understand-ing of and conformity to the moral principles of truth and justice.

8.2.1. Truth

Health care would simply not be possible if the people receiving care did not trust the people giving it. The recipient must believe in the truthfulness of the carer when she explains what is to be done, why and how. To tell the truth as part of a professional relationship seems such a basic requirement that it would seem to be unnecessary to explain it, and unthinkable to suggest that it is not always an absolute priority among the givers of health care.

Further investigation, however, reveals that it may not always be the accepted practice to tell the whole truth to a patient/client, demonstrating how the practice of a moral principle is not as straightforward as it first appears (Melia, 1987).

To tell the truth means giving a full and accurate account of the known facts of the situation: to accept the principle of truth is to accept an obligation to do this at all times. Where omission of information can distort the truth, what is not included in such an account may be just as important as what is included, so there are times when to withhold information means not telling the truth (Jones, 1989).

Examples of when this might happen include the following.

1. A poor prognosis may be kept from a patient with the justifi-cation that it is in his best interest to protect him from distress.
2. Possible but unlikely risks or side-effects of treatment may not be explained to a patient on the grounds that they will increase his anxiety unnecessarily.
3. Information concerning other people will not be repeated to a patient because it has been given in confidence.

In each of these situations the principle of truth has not been fully upheld. A moral decision has been made to override truth-telling as a guide to action when it is perceived to be to the advantage of the individual to withhold information from him.

When information is withheld, then by the nature of the decision the patient is not in a position to choose whether or not he agrees with it. He is unaware that he does not know all the facts, and he therefore cannot fully participate in decision-making about his care. Taken to extremes, this means that he has not agreed to receive the treatment given to him because he has not been truthfully told about it and is therefore receiving treatment, or being denied treatment, without consent and possibly against his will. Such action denies the principle of truth as well as the principle of autonomy.

The nurse should consider whether she finds the denial of these principles to be acceptable, and must be prepared to defend her actions and her patient's interest when a policy is chosen about giving him information. She must be able to explain the link between moral principles and particular actions in order to be able to justify her behaviour and therefore be accountable for it (Burnard and Chapman, 1988).

As with all other moral principles it would be comfortable to think that the principle of truth could be unconditionally relied upon in human interactions. Unfortunately, everyday practice reveals the difficulties that arise in seeking to attain this – as any other – moral principle. Principles are adapted to particular incidents; this flexibility and failure to make a complete match should not discourage the individual from seeking to meet as nearly as possible a match between action and beliefs.

8.2.2. Justice

Justice is another important principle to which a professional will conform. The relationship of trust between a profession and society depends on the professional exercising her expertise, for the good of that society, behaving justly toward those who need her expertise and being accountable for doing so. Justice concerns the organization of society and the ways the 'goods' of society are divided between individuals. The 'goods' include material resources, rights and privileges. Where justice is accepted by society, the way the 'goods' are distributed shows the translation of this principle into action. Justice may be served by dividing the 'goods' equally between all members of society, but clearly to give everyone the same of everything overlooks the differences between individuals in their needs and their values. It is normally accepted that justice is better served where 'goods' are divided unequally so that each member of society gets an unequal share of the 'goods' but the difference in what they receive relates to the differences in their needs and values. Rawls's Theory of Justice describes how the unequal division of 'goods' is just where the distribution does not disadvantage those who receive the least (Rawls, 1973).

The distribution of health care demands a commitment by society to the principle of justice. In the UK to date there remains a commitment to the ideals of the National Health Service where every individual is entitled to health care free at the point of delivery. People have an equal claim on the provision of health care where their needs are equal. However needs for health care are not equal so that justice is served where health care is provided unequally but people are treated differently according to differences in need. Complete conformity to this principle would demand that every individual were always given everything to maintain his health. Evidently, this does not describe what happens in practice. With the advances in science and technology in the twentieth century, the provision to every individual of everything he needs to maintain health is potentially limitless and could conceivably use up all the resources of even the wealthiest nation. It becomes necessary to seek to define the level of health which society considers that individuals have a right to expect and to allocate resources so as to reach that level. The principle of justice is challenged because of the huge potential for conflict concerning who can define health and health care needs, who should allocate resources and how they should be distributed (Melia, 1987). It must be decided whether justice is served if the cost and effectiveness of treatment is unequal. In this case it will be important to evaluate the treatment not in terms of equality but of equivalence. It must be recognized however that not only will cost and effectiveness vary objectively, but the perceived value of treatment to the individual will also vary – further complicating the calculation of equivalence.

In the interest of society, it should be expected that nurses, involved as they are in the delivery of health care, will understand the issues of these debates and will have given them careful and informed consideration.

Nurses are also involved in issues concerning the principle of justice on the more immediate level of daily practice when they allocate resources such as staff, time and materials (e.g., linen, dressings, toiletries).

Often it is physically impossible to meet every need of every patient, and it becomes inevitable that what is available must be divided. When this is the case, the nurse has to decide on priorities of care and must seek to exercise the principle of justice.

Justice is also served when the nurse respects the rights of each of her patients as an individual.

8.2.3. Patient/client interest

The second principle introducing the UKCC Code of Conduct is that the registered nurse shall 'safeguard the interest of the individual patient/client'.

This means that a nurse will provide physical safety for the individual, and will uphold and promote his interests – recognizing his right as an autonomous person. The moral principles underlying these behaviours are beneficence and autonomy.

Understanding moral principles is a professional responsibility. Logical, rational debate helps to guide behaviour when a course of action must be chosen. However, principles serve only as guidelines. As has been shown in the examples given, they cannot describe or decide on what should be done in particular instances. They do not function, for example, in the same way as an anatomy reference book which can provide answers by giving factual information. What they can do is to allow a systematic evaluation of the alternatives so that a choice is made with a clear understanding of underlying beliefs.

Jonathan Glover (1984) suggests that the social function of the study of ethics is: 'To spell out different sets of values more fully than they usually appear, so that people can accept or reject policies with a greater awareness of the implications of their choices.'

8.2.4. Physical safety

Maintenance of the physical environment where care is given is to some extent outside the control of the staff nurse. She is dependent on others, for example, for the provision of resources (including staff, clean linen, and meals), the maintenance of equipment and cleaning services.

Where conditions are such that a staff nurse considers them unsuitable for the provision of care she faces a moral decision in choosing whether to give or withhold care in such circumstances. If she gives care she may know that to do so exposes her patient to a degree of risk. For example, she may know that there are not enough staff to evacuate the ward in the event of fire; that the junior students working in the ward are inadequately supervised; that the bedpan machine is faulty; that there are not enough clean pyjamas in the ward for patients to change as required.

But if she chooses not to give care, perhaps while insisting that improvements are made, she is also failing to promote some aspects of patient safety when the patient is in immediate need of a particular treatment.

These are examples of the moral decisions that a staff nurse is called upon to make every day.

The UKCC offers guidelines to help her to choose her course of action in such situations. One clear guideline states that 'The nurse will work in a collaborative and cooperative manner with other health care professionals.' (UKCC Code of Conduct: Clause 5). In this case the hospital management share with her the responsibility for the physical environment.

Another guideline states, 'Practitioners on the Register will ensure that the reality of their clinical environment is made known to and understood by the appropriate authorities' (UKCC *Exercising Accountability* p. 9). This recognizes that the nurse does not have total overall control over the environment where she works, and in making known the realities of that environment she can expect cooperation in improving conditions.

The nurse is also responsible for maintaining the patient's safety in her delivery of nursing care. Nursing treatments will be chosen and implemented based on nursing expertise; particularly where primary nursing is practised the nurse will be responsible for deciding which treatment to carry out and for implementing and evaluating the treatment.

Nurses also participate in medical treatment, for example giving medication prescribed by medical staff, preparing patients for medical treatment and assisting with medical treatment. In this area of nursing practice the nurse will probably not be directly involved in deciding on the treatment she participates in, and this can raise a moral dilemma if she does not agree with the chosen treatment.

When a nurse does not agree with a course of action chosen by the health care team she works with she has to make a moral decision. She may choose not to participate in the care of the patients, although she must ensure that this does not threaten the patient's safety, or she may decide to override her personal views so that the care given to a patient follows a consistent policy although not the one she considers to be right. To make this choice means choosing between personal and professional standards and must be done with a clear understanding of the underlying ethical issues. Whichever course she chooses she is still responsible for her actions, if she chooses to participate in treatment she does not pass her responsibility on to those whose decisions she is implementing. A nurse needs courage to express her beliefs in this situation, but it is important that she does so; to deny her moral dilemma can be a major source of stress.

There are two guidelines from the UKCC which may help a nurse to reach her decision: in the UKCC Code of Professional Conduct, Clause 7 states that the nurse shall 'make known to an appropriate person or authority any conscientious objection which may be relevant to professional practice'; while Clause 5, as previously quoted, states that she will 'work in a collaborative and cooperative manner with other health care professionals'.

Relating the guidelines to specific situations in practice should help the practitioner to identify right behaviour.

8.3. Safeguarding the patient's/client's interests

This assumes the principle of benevolence (well-wishing), where any action taken by the health care team is directed to the patient/client's best interest. Actions are taken because it is considered that the outcomes of these actions are more to the advantage of the client than would be the outcomes of any alternative actions. Problems arise in identifying which are the patient's best interests.

Generally, health care professionals are concerned to promote health and prolong life, and it would seem reasonable to suppose that they will be acting in the patient's best interest if they do so; but this may not always be the case. Depending on what definition of 'health' is accepted it may be argued that there are occasions when a patient can be kept healthy but derive no benefit from it.

1. A patient with a chronic disease may find the treatment an unbearable burden.
2. A brain dead patient on a ventilator may have an otherwise perfectly functioning 'healthy' body.

Similarly it may not always be in the patient's best interest to prolong his life, e.g., painful palliative surgery to prolong life by a few months may not be in the patient's best interest.

These simple examples demonstrate clearly that it is necessary to think more carefully about what it really means to safeguard the patient's best interest, because best interest extends beyond mere physical survival to include considerations of the quality of life.

Health care professionals, in taking decisions about treatment, are called upon to evaluate the quality of someone else's life. This is obviously an extremely difficult task. The decision making is further complicated by the facts that not only is the outcome of health care inevitably uncertain, but also each individual's response to the outcome is impossible to predict. Evaluating the benefits to be derived from particular treatments is a formidable responsibility. There is also the option to withhold treatment if this is considered to be in the patient's best interest, for instance, when a frail elderly patient with a dense hemiparesis is not given antibiotics when he develops pneumonia, and in this case to choose not to act is to take a positive ethical stance.

The patient may or may not be involved in the decision-making process; deciding whether or not to include him may constitute part of the decision to be made. This may raise a moral dilemma where decisions based on expertise override the patient's right of self-determination: such behaviour is known as paternalism. (See also, informed consent, discussed below.)

Fundamental to the understanding of the ethical aspects of nursing practice is the recognition of moral principles that underlie action and are based on the values, attitudes and beliefs of society.

8.4. Legal aspects of care

The legal code describes standards of behaviour which are demanded of the individual by society, and are therefore more clearly stated than are moral standards. Legal standards derive either from a tradition of practice (common law) or from decisions made by parliament (statute law) and can be enforced through courts of law.

There are some differences between the law in England and Wales and the law in Scotland: in terminology, in practice and in the organization of the law courts. It is the responsibility of the nurse to be aware of her legal position in whichever country she works – ignorance is no defence in law.

The law governs behaviour in two ways. Criminal law defines behaviour which is considered to be socially unacceptable and may be related to the state (e.g., treason), the person (e.g., homicide) or property (e.g., theft).

The purpose of criminal law is that the values of society be maintained. Where they are contravened penalties can be exacted varying in severity according to society's perception of the seriousness of the crime and on what it considers to be the purpose of punishment.

Civil law concerns dispute between individuals, where the behaviour itself may be harmless, but on certain occasions it may cause unfair disadvantages to other people. It includes the following.

1. The law of tort – or delict in Scotland (wrong, or harm to another, e.g., libel, slander).
2. The law of contract (concerning agreed terms of employment etc.).
3. The law of persons (relating to individuals' rights).
4. The law of succession (concerning wills and gifts).

Its aim is to promote justice for individuals in society.

The nurse has obligations in law both as an individual and as a professional practitioner. Her obligations as an individual are the same as those of any other member of society, but as a professional practitioner she has additional obligations to conform to the code of conduct of her profession, being answerable both in law and to her profession to do so.

The nursing profession is recognized in law and therefore has certain rights and responsibilities. It has a legal right to control entry to the profession and a responsibility to establish a code of professional conduct (a code of ethics) for its members. Membership of the nursing profession (i.e., registration) is controlled by the UKCC in that it sets the criteria for entry to a recognized training institution, the content, method and standard of the education and training given there and the standard of knowledge and expertise considered appropriate for nursing practice and by association for admission to the register at the end of training.

It is recognized in law that the UKCC will make these decisions, and only those people whose names are on the Register may legally use the title 'nurse'.

Registered nurses agree to abide by the UKCC code of professional conduct, which conformity allows the profession to meet its responsibility to uphold agreed standards of conduct. In this way, through control of entry by the profession being recognized in law, the profession is able to ensure that public interest is served, in that anyone legitimately using the title 'nurse' will uphold the code of conduct.

It should be noted that a student nurse is permitted as a courtesy, to use the title 'nurse' at work, but would be misrepresenting her status should she claim the title in any other context.

Legal issues which are of professional concern to the staff nurse and to which she should therefore give consideration include the following.

1. Her contract of employment: including termination, dismissal and disciplinary procedures.
2. Documentation.
3. Confidentiality.
4. Patient's consent.
5. Negligence.

8.4.1. The contract of employment

On taking up employment as a registered nurse, it is normally required that a contract be drawn up by the employer and signed by the employee in order to state the terms under which the nurse is employed.

As with all legal documents there are precise requirements of what must be included in a contract of employment in order for it to be valid in law. It must specify between whom the contract has been made, i.e., naming the employee and the employer, and it must specify the terms of employment related to the hours to be worked, salary, entitlement to sick pay and holidays and the period of notice required on either side to terminate the contract. The contract binds both the employer and the employee to the terms that it describes. If any information in the contract, or any information as a result of which the contract was offered is found to be false, the contract is no longer valid and there is no requirement on either side to continue with the employment.

It should be noted with regard to the employment of nurses that because of the nature of their work they are obliged to declare details of previous convictions. This is required by the Rehabilitation of Offenders Act 1974, Exemptions Order 1975, and enables the employer to protect the public where it might be considered that the nature of a previous conviction indicates that a particular individual might be seen to be unsuitable for employment as a nurse.

A contract may be open (with no time-limit) or it may be for a fixed term. It may specify the number of hours to be worked without detailing when they will be rostered, and it may specify a hospital rather than a particular ward or area where the nurse will be required to work. Such details will be made clear in the contract, and by signing the contract the nurse accepts the conditions it describes. She is obliged to honour the terms of her contract and makes a legal commitment to do so when she signs it. She also has an obligation to her profession to accept the responsibilities of practice. Health employers will normally issue job descriptions and policies and procedures for practice all of which guide the actions of the employee and incorporate legal requirements such as Health and Safety at Work, the Mental Health Act and the Control of Medicines Act.

These policies, together with the theory base indicated by the nurse's professional status, ensure that the nurse is able to fulfil the requirements of the job, which she has legally bound herself to do when she signs a contract of employment.

Conditions governing the termination of a contract will be explicit in the contract so that it can be simply and legally terminated where these conditions are met. Either the employer or the employee would be in breach of contract if they disregard the conditions of termination of employment in the contract. There is also a legal process for the dismissal of an employee should she be guilty of general or gross misconduct.

Examples of misconduct include the following.

1. Theft from hospital or patients.
2. Errors in drug administration.
3. Inadequate care for patient safety.
4. Poor attendance at work.

When dismissing a nurse, the employer is required by law to follow the correct disciplinary procedure, as shown in Fig. 8.2.

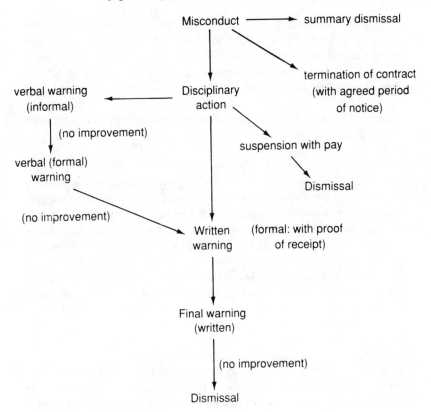

Figure 8.2 Flow chart leading to dismissal

The employer must be able to justify his actions, and show that he has given adequate warning to the employee; and the nurse has a legal right of appeal.

Being accountable to her profession as well as to her employer, it is likely that if a nurse is the subject of disciplinary or legal action she will also be called to answer to her profession for her conduct. The disciplinary procedure of the UKCC will function independently of legal or employment-related actions, and the profession will exact its own penalties regardless of any decision made by the employer or the law. For example, theft of a small quantity of medicines of little monetary value may not be severely penalized in law but could be considered by the UKCC to justify removal from the Register of the nurse found guilty of the theft. In this case the penalty exacted by the UKCC can have more serious implications than the outcome of legal procedures for the nurse. The UKCC acts within the law but on occasions conduct being judged may assume greater or less significance when seen in the context of professional practice, and the outcome of UKCC disciplinary procedures can be more or less severe than the outcome in law.

Behaviours in which the nurse has responsibilities in law include the following.

Documentation
The requirement in law to state explicitly all relevant details as described in the drawing up of a contract of employment applies equally to any written record which can be used in legal proceedings. It therefore applies to all written nursing records. Any documentation which records treatment given, patient condition and progress may be used to establish the facts of a particular situation or event. Investigations may take place long after it occurred, so written records are extremely important in establishing what was happening to a particular patient (or nurse) at a particular time.

Written records include the following.

Medicine Administration Chart.
This documents medication given to a patient, the dosage, the time and date and the identity of the nurses responsible. It must be completed after the patient has taken the medicine, because it records the administration not the prescription of the medication. Should the patient refuse prescribed medication (as he is entitled to do), or should there be any other reason why medication is not given this must be recorded on the chart.

Nursing care plans
Nursing notes are not legal documents but may be used during legal procedures to establish the facts of a case, e.g., the condition of a patient at a particular time and what was done for him.

It is therefore important that nursing records use clear, unambiguous language, giving an accurate account of what is to be recorded, avoiding abbreviations which may be misunderstood or even not understood at all, and avoiding opinion and inference. All nursing charts will be kept and may be used for reference. Where primary nursing is practised it is particularly important that records are kept accurately to detail care given, because the nurse initiates

care and is accountable for her actions. She must have a clear record of the decisions she has made and the care she has given.

Incident forms

An incident form is completed when an accident or incident occurs and either a member of staff, a patient or another person is injured. The form provides a written record of the sequence of events and must therefore give a detailed and accurate account. Diagrams may help and can be used to supplement the information given. The incident form, like other written records, may be used at any time (often a considerable time after the event) to establish what happened.

Witnesses to the accident or injury will be asked to give their names and addresses and to sign the incident form. The injured party will be advised to seek medical advice (or will be seen by a doctor if a patient). A report of the injury will be kept, as will a record of action taken subsequent to the event, e.g., changes in practice or, disciplinary action.

The completed incident form is kept by the hospital administration department if a staff member or other person is involved, or the medical administration department, when a patient is involved; and it may be used for reference if an individual seeks compensation for industrial injury or as a result of violence or negligence.

It should be noted that an employer is not liable for injury at work (e.g., back injury) when it is the result of bad practice (e.g., unsafe lifting) and it is established that teaching has been given regarding that practice (safe lifting is taught as part of the preparation for registration of nurses). The employer is also not liable if it can be seen that he has provided proper tools and a safe system of work. Similarly in cases of violence and negligence, an employer need only show that he has provided a safe environment within reasonable limits to be free of liability. It would be useful for a staff nurse to familiarize herself with the Health and Safety at Work Acts.

Nurses' reports

A staff nurse in the NHS has a teaching commitment and is required to make a written assessment of the progress of student nurses she works with. In doing this the staff nurse has responsibilities both to the student nurse (to assess and encourage progress), and to her profession (to maintain standards of practice).

Satisfactory clinical reports during training are necessary for the successful completion of training, and therefore for registration.

A staff nurse's report must give a fair and truthful appraisal of the student nurse's ability, and if the student nurse's work is not considered satisfactory the staff nurse has a responsibility to make this known. A report written honestly, without malice and by a person whose duty it is to make it, is not subject to the law of defamation (libel) so the staff nurse's report must satisfy these criteria for her report to be acceptable in law.

A report indicating that a student is considered unsafe to practice can lead to termination of training. When this is the case it must be shown that the student has been given adequate warning (similar to the informal warning in a disciplinary action) to give her the opportunity to improve and this will take the form of ongoing clinical assessment.

Such action (the termination of employment) can only be taken as a result of a report which clearly states that the student's clinical practice is unsafe. It is crucial therefore that the staff nurse be able to justify her criticisms and be prepared to express them in such a situation.

All written records must show the date of recording, and where relevant they must be signed. (This does not necessarily apply to nursing charts.) Should the need to make corrections on written records arise, Tipp-Ex may not be used and a correction must be made, using a single line to score through incorrect information.

Above all it is important that any information recorded in writing in the course of nursing practice would bear scrutiny in a court of law.

Related to the legal implications of the documentation of information is the issue of confidentiality of information. Legal and ethical considerations are relevant in considering how a professional nurse should act in this regard.

8.4.2. Confidentiality and informed consent

This is further elaborated upon in the UKCC advisory document, *Confidentiality*, which states that a registered nurse, midwife and health visitor shall 'respect confidential information obtained in the course of professional practice and refrain from disclosing such information without the consent of the patient/client, or a person entitled to act on his/her behalf, except where disclosure is

required by law or by the order of a court or is in the public interest'. This makes it clear that information given to a nurse must be held in confidence, and that breaches in confidence must only occur when there is good reason for them. Disclosure of information can occur in the following circumstances.

1. In law: the law does not allow anyone giving evidence to withhold information on the grounds that it is confidential.
2. With the patient's consent.
3. When it is considered by the individual nurse using her professional judgement to be in the public interest, e.g., when the nurse becomes aware that the patient is involved in serious crime.
4. By accident, which constitutes professional misconduct.

A nurse is also responsible for ensuring that written information about her patients is kept safely and in such a way as to maintain the confidence of the patients concerned. Written records must be kept in secure and private storage. The patient is entitled to see his own records where they are stored on computer, under the Data Protection Act (1984), but as the law stands at present there is no requirement that he have access to written records. Although information is kept safely in confidence, it is obviously important that it is effectively communicated to everyone involved in care of the patient where it is relevant for the carer in her relationship with the patient.

With the increase of computerised record-keeping comes an increasing need for examination of the issues of confidentiality. Computers must be used in such a way that relevant information is available to staff and to the patient himself, but remains protected from unauthorized computer users.

The legal requirement concerning confidentiality is clear; the nurse has a duty to keep information in confidence, whether it is given verbally or in writing, because individual privacy is an important concept in law. She also has a duty to part with such information should she be required to do so in the course of legal proceedings, and will be committing perjury should she fail in this duty – her legal duty is to give information, regardless of its confidential nature, given as it was within a professional relationship. Knowing this, there may be occasions when a nurse feels it right to warn a patient of the legal position regarding information before he discloses it to her.

Ethically, there is more potential for a dilemma to arise: where information is not required by law the nurse may still have reason to decide that a breach in confidentiality serves the public interest, regardless of her commitment to the underlying principle of confidentiality. (This may occur, for example, if the nurse becomes aware that the patient intends to harm another person.)

Information may be divulged for legal or for ethical reasons, it may also be divulged with the patient's consent. For example, a patient may agree to make his diagnosis known to another patient with the same diagnosis, at the nurse's suggestion, so that they could discuss their situation to their mutual advantage. The patient will decide whether or not to follow this course of action, in the same way that he can decide whether to agree or refuse any form of treatment or intervention.

8.4.3. Patient consent

A patient must give consent, and therefore has the right to refuse consent for any treatment offered to him.

Consent is not required in certain situations regulated by the Mental Health Acts, and there are situations where consent may be given by the next of kin, for example, on behalf of an unconscious person, a child or a person of unsound mind. However, for a patient of sound mind, treatment (e.g., the administration of prescribed medicines) cannot be given legally without consent; if it is this constitutes assault and battery, and whoever gave the treatment may be sued for damages.

Consent can be implied or formal. Implied consent is when the patient's consent is indicated in his acceptance of treatment; the fact that he has been admitted to hospital, has stayed there and has cooperated in his care implies that he consents to the treatment he receives. Formal consent is given in response to direct requests from those giving treatment for permission to proceed, and the consent is given either verbally or in writing, e.g., by signing a consent form.

The difficulty in asking for patient consent is in ensuring that he is giving informed consent. To give informed consent, the patient must be physically and psychologically in a condition to do so, and must have adequate knowledge and understanding of the options, the risks and the expected outcome either to choose which of several treatment options to take, or to choose whether or not to accept treatment. Treatment cannot be given without consent and it is the responsibility of the people offering the treatment to ensure that the patient is sufficiently well informed for the consent he gives to be meaningful.

The doctor is responsible for getting consent for medical treatment such as the signing of a consent form for a surgical procedure. The nurse, involved as she is in preparing the patient for medical treatment as well as delivering nursing care, is responsible for ensuring that her patient has consented to receive the care that she offers. If he refuses his consent, she must, legally and morally, respect his wishes. The issue of informed consent is an extensive and complex subject – readers are recommended to consider the matter further (Faulder, 1985).

Once a patient has consented to receive treatment the nurse has a duty of care to that patient. In taking care of her patients, a nurse is personally responsible for maintaining standards to the level of her competence (i.e., within her own field of practice) and can be sued for negligence if she fails in this duty.

To prove negligence in law, three points must be established.

1. It must be shown that the person claiming to have suffered from negligence had a right to expect care

   (the carer was under a duty of care).

2. It must be shown that the care given was inadequate

   (that there was a breach in that duty).

3. It must be shown that the suffering was caused by the failure in care

   (that the damage resulted from a breach of care).

Examples of negligence in nursing care include, for instance, scalding a patient in a hot bath or, giving incorrect medication.

In each of these cases, the nurse was under a duty of care to her patient, a patient has a right to expect help with bathing and accurate administration of medication from a nurse.

In each case, the nurse failed in her duty to give the care safely – she did not check the temperature of the water or the medication, which it was reasonable to expect that she would do; and as a result of her failure of care, the patient suffered injury – was scalded, or was at risk from the wrong medication or the wrong dose.

As well as being liable for her own actions at work, the staff nurse is also responsible when she delegates work to others. Her duty of care is such that it is her responsibility that patients receive care even when she does not directly give that care herself. If it can be shown that nursing work has been inappropriately delegated, for example, if junior nurses have been asked to undertake tasks which they are not sufficiently skilled to do, and have not been taught or supervised in undertaking these tasks, then the nurse delegating work is responsible for negligence. She has failed in her duty of care by not making provision for care to be given safely.

While the nurse is accountable for giving and organizing care within her sphere of competence, her employer also has a responsibility to give her adequate and appropriate support so that she can fulfil her duty of care. The employer has the responsibility to provide a safe and suitable environment of care and to ensure that his staff are appropriately prepared to work in that environment. He has a responsibility to provide the necessary teaching, supervision and support of his staff, just as nurses have the responsibility to take advantage of such provision to develop their professional competence according to their needs.

Employer and employee share responsibility in the provision of care. A nurse is personally liable for her actions within her sphere of competence, but her employer accepts vicarious liability for his employees. When a patient sues for damages following negligence, (which, if he does, he must do within three years of the incident) it is usual for him to sue the employer rather than the individual employee. The employer can then take action against the employee and the nurse will also be answerable to the UKCC – her professional body.

Outside her working environment, the nurse is still accountable for her actions. If called to use her professional skills and knowledge in any situation the nurse must recognize her position in law. If she assumes a duty of care for an individual (e.g., following a road traffic accident) should the care she gives – **within the limitation of her competence** – be inadequate and cause harm, she will be considered to be negligent. If she fails to give care when she would have been able to give it, and it is considered that she had a duty of care on that particular occasion, she will also be considered negligent.

Litigation relating to health care is increasing, and nurses as professional practitioners have a responsibility both to themselves and to their profession to understand how they should act according to the law.

The UKCC is legally recognized by the Nurses, Midwives and Health Visitors Act (1979) as being responsible for promoting and improving standards of professional conduct. It does this by controlling entry to the profession and by calling practitioners to account for their actions. The UKCC has issued guidelines explaining the conduct required of professional nurses, midwives and health visitors. It is expected that members of the profession will behave in accordance with these guidelines and to do so, the individual practitioner needs to have an understanding of the moral implications and the legal requirements of her practice (Ryden *et al.*, 1989).

It is hoped that the aspects discussed in this chapter have helped to outline what some of these implications and requirements are, have been of interest and will help staff nurses entering the profession.

References

Beauchamps, T. and Childress, J. (1983) *Biomedical Ethics* OUP, Oxford.

Burnard, P., and Chapman, C. (1988) *Professional and Ethical Issues in Nursing*, John Wiley and Sons, Chichester.

Faulder, C. (1985) *Whose Body Is It?*, Virago, London.

Glover, J. (1984) *What Sort of People Should There Be?*, Penguin, Harmondsworth.

Hull, R. (1980) *Responsibility and Accountability Analysed, Nursing Outlook*, Dec, pp. 707–12.

Jones, C. (1989) Little White Lies, *Nursing Times* Nov, 85, 44, pp. 38–9.

Melia, K. (1987) Everyday Ethics for Nurses, *Nursing Times* Jan, 83, 3, pp. 28–30.

Melia, K. (1987) Everyday Ethics for Nurses, *Nursing Times* June, 83, 25, pp. 42–4.

Pyne, R. (1988) On Being Accountable, *Health Visitor*, June, 61 pp. 173–6.

Rawls, J. (1973) *A Theory of Justice*, OUP, Oxford.

Ryden, M.B. *et al.* (1989) Wrestling with the Larger Picture: Placing ethical behaviour in context, *Journal of Nursing Education*, June, 28, 6 pp 271–5.

Schrock, R. (1990) Conscience and Courage: A critical examination of professional conduct, *Nurse Education Today* 10, pp. 3–9.

Skerry, R. (1983) *Science and Moral Priority*, Blackwell, Oxford.

UKCC (1984) *Code of Professional Conduct for the Nurse, Midwife and Health Visitor*, UKCC, London.

UKCC (1987) *Confidentiality* UKCC, London.

UKCC (1989) *Exercising Accountability*, UKCC, London.

Young, A. (1981) *Legal Problems in Nursing Practice*, Lippincott, Philadelphia.

9

Effective use of resources

Rose Fleming

9.1. Introduction

'Money, money, money', 'Money makes the world go round', 'Money is the root of all evil.' I would like to suggest that money is the resource which is essential to all aspects of patient care and is the common denominator in the 'Five Ms' of management – manpower; materials; machinery; methods; money.

Since the beginning of the National Health Service in 1948 the cost of health care has continually escalated. In 1949, it cost £414 million – 3.95% of the gross domestic product, in 1982 this had risen to £10 856 million – 6.2% of the GDP and the projected cost for 1990/91 is £20 830 million (HMSO, 1989).

In the 1960s when medical knowledge and technology were taking off, money was, by today's standards, easily available. Provided advancement or improvement in patient care could be demonstrated, funding was usually available and replacements were guaranteed on presentation of the old or damaged article. Halcyon days indeed! However, the financial problems of the 1970s and the changes in the country's oil industry brought this comfortable, privileged position of the caring professions to an end.

In addition to the political and financial pressures, the Health Service has had to come to terms with the demographic changes, and a consumer who is not only more aware of what is available, but is more demanding and critical of the service provided. To compound the problem, the increase in new treatments available has not, to any large extent, been matched by a decline in demand for others.

Changes in legislation have in many instances increased the financial burden of managers. For example, the lifting of Crown Immunity (G.M. Bath, 1985) and the accompanying protection of Crown employees has, in many health establishments, required considerable expenditure to meet the Health and Safety requirements (HMSO, 1974).

Never before has it been so important for nurse managers to manage every aspect of their resources effectively. Like general management the management of resources can be addressed under the headings of the Five Ms.

9.2. Manpower – human resources

Human resources are the most costly item in the Health Service budget, accounting for 70% of the total expenditure, and nursing accounts for approximately 45% of the total manpower in the NHS (Raybould, 1977).

It is therefore inevitable that the nursing work force is given special attention when funding is limited or contracting, for by reducing manpower there is perceived to be a guaranteed saving in expenditure. The importance of creating accurate and realistic nursing establishments cannot be over-emphasized. For too long the number of nurses assumed to be needed was based on historical concepts and shift patterns. Practices were not questioned, new procedures were often just absorbed into the system – 'creeping developments' – until too late the cry of staffing implications fell on deaf ears.

Alternatively, every change was met with a demand for more staff, resulting in many having a sceptical attitude towards the way nurses managed their manpower resources.

In recent years many new methods have been developed to calculate nursing establishments. In Scotland there has been an attempt to standardize manpower levels by encouraging the use of just two tools – the Aberdeen Formula (1969) and the Telford System (1983).

The Aberdeen Formula is possibly the more scientific in its application, by initially utilizing a twenty-eight day assessment of patient dependency for ward areas. It also takes formal account of influencing factors including ward layout, technical nursing levels, administrative tasks and support services. However, in practice it has proved more appropriate for acute areas.

The Telford System is perhaps more subjective in its approach, starting with an assessment of manpower needs by the charge nurses and nurse managers responsible for the area concerned. In practice this system is perceived to be more sympathetic to the care of long-term and chronically ill patients.

No matter which method is chosen (and others are being developed in the light of previous experience), accurate results are dependent on the nurses involved using truly professional judgement and expertise in their assessment of all aspects of the analysis. Professional responsibility and judgement do not end with the initial exercises of these methods. Good manpower planning should result in achieving set objectives on the care of a number of patients, with the most appropriately skilled staff in sufficient numbers to ensure the safety of both patients and staff. Therefore, in establishing the number of staff required skill-mix must be taken into account, and indeed it may be more cost effective to reduce qualified staff in some areas, and increase them in others. In addition to the use of part-time staff, job sharing should be seriously considered, especially in view of the projected fall in the available manpower, particularly the reduction in school leavers.

Before leaving the subject of who should perform different activities, thought must be given to the mix of male and female staff to account for the patients' needs and preferences. Having identified the staff required and the skills they need to achieve the objectives of a ward or department, the other aspects of manpower management must be addressed. These include the following.

1. The recruitment of staff.
2. The maintenance of staff skills and their standards.
3. The retention of staff.
4. The re-employment of registered nurses after a career break.

The recruitment of staff is the first step towards building a strong, cohesive, amicable team. When selecting new members, thought must be given to matching the person with not only the job, but also with those already working in the ward or department. It is often easier to train people to new procedures and policies than to change their attitudes and personalities. It is not unknown for a new member of staff to disrupt a previously happy, efficient ward.

Selection is a difficult exercise, for while there are books and courses to help those concerned to improve their ability, practical experience is essential to identify the different approaches and techniques of both interviewer and interviewee. Even with considerable experience it is quite possible to err in the choice, especially with those who can sell themselves well. It is also worth noting that it is easier to employ a person than to discharge one. However, if time and trouble are taken in the preparation work identifying the type of person required, their skills, and the objectives of the post and department, careful interviewing should result in a good match even if some early training of the successful candidate is required.

Retention of staff is perhaps even more difficult than recruitment. Most staff will remain in post provided they are happy, obtain job satisfaction from their work and their domestic or social circumstances do not change. Realistically, the employer alone cannot achieve this, but they should provide the environment and experience for the staff to maintain their skills and standards. With a good creative approach to the appraisal system and quality control tools, much can be done to assist nursing staff to feel fulfilled.

Of particular importance is the need to maintain and further the knowledge and ability of the nurse. In addition to the opportunities to learn in the clinical areas, there are now a wide variety of teaching aids. If these are not available from the Colleges of Nursing the material most appropriate to the current clinical practice is often available from an alternative source, e.g., commercial companies or library films. In conjunction with tutorials from other professionals, in-service training can assist all grades of staff to improve their care and understanding of patients. However, time is the scarce element and this shortcoming can only be overcome with determination and good planning. I would suggest that a regular tutorial once each month which takes place and is interesting, is better than a programme of weekly sessions, 75% of which have to be cancelled.

This professional development of staff, both academically and clinically requires careful planning to ensure not only that members of staff progress in their chosen field, but also that service to patients is maintained. The English National Board Courses and in Scotland, Professional Studies (PS) Modules have assisted nurses to achieve higher standards of care and management. Equally the concept of formal, ongoing training should ensure staff keep up with advances in medical practice and nursing care. While acknowledging that some educationalists still have much to overcome to achieve recognition for Post Registration Courses, those in the clinical areas must recognize their considerable responsibilities towards the realization of this tuition and training for registered nurses.

It has been suggested that advancement on the career ladder is not, for many, the vital factor. A research project undertaken at the Royal Marsden Hospital, London (Tiffney, 1984), in which the nurse's role has been formally broadened to include clinician, educationalist, researcher and manager, has demonstrated that staff turnover is reduced when nurses find their work both challenging and fulfilling. Projects in other Regions have lent weight to this theory (Pearson, 1988 and Purdy *et al.*, 1988). Nevertheless, with the anticipated nationwide shortage of staff, due to the fall in school leavers noted earlier, it will be those who can provide the facilities to achieve both professional and job satisfaction who will retain their staff.

The re-employment of registered nurses who have taken a career break, normally to care for their children, is not a new concept, but in the future it will become vital to sustain the levels of trained nurses required (Clay 1987). Potential employees from the many unemployed nurses – it is said the loss is 35% (Clay, 1987) – frequently lack confidence in their own ability and potential due to the speed at which modern medicine and treatments are perceived to progress. 'Back to Nursing' courses outlining the main aspects of current nursing practice and presented in a manner which is attractive, logical and stimulating can do much to overcome such anxieties. Likewise the knowledge that good orientation programmes on beginning employment, geared to the actual position the nurse will occupy, will further encourage the return of these valuable members of the community.

Finally, a good manager of personnel should consider each member of staff, as one should the patient, as a whole person. In this, thought must be given to her personal needs, as an individual and often as part of a family unit. For instance, in accepting part-time staff with young families, the manager must also accept there may be a family crisis and no child minder available. A degree of flexibility and perceived fairness in all aspects of staff management is essential. Equally staff must recognize that employment is a joint contract with commitment and responsibilities on both sides. With this philosophy respected, good staff morale can be achieved along with adequate staffing and high standards of care.

9.3. Materials

Nurses are one of the few groups of staff involved in providing a full twenty-four hour service in health care, and since they account for 45% of the NHS workforce (Raybould, 1977), their potential influence on day-to-day expenditure, even disregarding salaries, is unquestionable. However, the registered nurses' opportunities to affect the use of resources almost doubles when it is recognized that they control the activities of nursing auxiliaries, students and pupil nurses, who make up 41% of the working establishment – 24% and 17% respectively. In addition, the trained nurse can have considerable influence on other groups of staff who look to nursing staff for the provision of materials and equipment to carry out treatments and other duties.

Many materials used by nurses and other health carers are those traditionally accepted in an institution or chosen by others for cost-saving purposes. Often insufficient thought and discussion with the users takes place and the users, while complaining of the quality or suitability, provide insufficient evidence to implement change. Nevertheless, the savings which can be effected by the wise use of materials are frequently underestimated. It is these savings which are perhaps the real economies which should be emphasized to all health carers.

Materials and sundries fall into two main groups; those which are directly associated with patient care, e.g., catheters, sutures, incontinence aids etc., and those indirectly affecting patients, such as hand towels, staff uniforms, cleaning materials. While in the assessment of any product the questions are similar, the emphasis is somewhat different.

The first consideration in selecting any materials or sundries directly involved in patient care must be, do they achieve the original objective in a safe and timely manner with no side-effects to either the patient or staff? Another aspect in the selection of materials is the suitability of presentation to allow the nurse to adhere to an accepted procedure, e.g., an aseptic technique, in any given situation. The procedure requires the article to be sterile at the point of use, but by virtue of the materials available, and its assembly and method of presentation, it is almost impossible to effect a clean, sterile product, e.g., sachets of cleansing fluids. Alternatively some sundries are not available for lengthy periods during servicing, e.g., those sent for ethylene oxide sterilization cannot be used until five days after exposure to allow all the gas to be dissipated.

Such restrictions in the flexibility of use are not only time-consuming for nurses in arranging reprocessing, but can limit the extent of patient care. It is therefore essential that nursing staff take an active professional attitude towards the selection and purchase of materials to be used in their fields of care. Thus nurses can ensure the most appropriate items are purchased while in many instances effecting real savings. After selection the savings begin with the method of purchase, i.e., on contract or in such quantities, if storage allows, to warrant a percentage discount from the supplier, hence the advantage of central stores.

It is often items involved in indirect patient care which can attract considerable savings. In one instance, by changing the supplier of hand towels used by operating theatre staff, an annual saving of £9000–£10 000 was achieved (Lothian, 1988). The towel, although slightly smaller, was effective and the standard of aseptic technique maintained. Initial trials, before establishing an annual arrangement with the supplier, ensured the majority of users found the new product acceptable. Choosing an intravenous catheter or similar product, directly affecting the patient, requires much greater care in the function and safety aspects, and without doubt the medical staff would be involved. Nevertheless, as with any disposable product there is the potential for considerable savings, and it is here that nursing staff can encourage good practice.

This conscientious use of materials and sundries commences with selecting the right item for the procedure in hand, also the right size and the correct amount. Taking a single-use catheter too big or too small, through bad initial assessment of need, can result in a financial loss of between £1.00 to £12.00 on each occasion. Annually this type of saving can be significant.

Similarly, encouraging nursing and other staff to economize on the quantity of items used can result in considerable efficiencies, this includes suture materials, cleaning materials and dressings.

Other choices requiring careful assessment are those comparing single-use or disposable goods with re-usable equivalents. In making a valid judgement there are three main considerations – performance and suitability for the procedure (perhaps the most important), safety and cost. While the first two, performance and safety, may be quite clear, the assessment of cost can be more difficult. The cost of a single-use item is straightforward, but account must still be taken of the manpower involved in purchasing and transporting it safely to the point of use. For re-usable items the costing is more complex, as the whole recycling process must be considered, including materials, overheads, transport, labour and administrative costs. In certain circumstances a sliding scale is required to make appropriate charges (Table 9.1. Ethylene Oxide Charges). In other instances it is necessary to include a depreciation charge if the reprocessing unit is responsible for replacing worn or broken items.

The size of the sterilizer chamber determines the amount of gas required and an indicator is used for each cycle. The cost of these are therefore standard for every cycle – the fixed costs.

To calculate the cost of each item sterilized, the fixed cost is divided by the number of items in the cycle and added to the cost of packaging – the variable cost. The total price includes 15% VAT plus an administrative charge.

Table 9.1. Ethylene oxide sterilization and packing

No. of packs sterilized in the cycle	Fixed cost £	Variable cost £	Total cost £	Net unit cost £	Gross unit cost (per pack) £
1	5.52	.44	5.96	5.96	6.56
5	5.52	2.20	7.72	1.54	1.70
10	5.52	4.40	9.92	.99	1.09
20	5.52	8.80	14.32	.72	.79
30	5.52	13.20	18.72	.62	.69
40	5.52	17.60	23.12	.58	.64
50	5.52	22.00	27.52	.55	.61
60	5.52	26.40	31.92	.53	.59
70	5.52	30.80	36.32	.52	.57
80	5.52	35.20	40.72	.51	.56
90	5.52	39.60	45.12	.50	.55
100	5.52	44.00	49.52	.50	.54

Because of Government pressures on Health Service managers to make the NHS function within its budget, product selection panels have to choose commodities for patient care with cost as one of their priorities. In this situation the user's opinion on the suitability of a product becomes essential if effective and safe patient care is to be achieved. However, their case must be backed with valid judgements, good information and hard data. Nursing staff, not least, must ensure they play their role in obtaining the best cost-effective materials and sundries to care for their patients to a high standard.

Choices made carefully after realistic trials can be very effective in preventing an apparent saving becoming quite the opposite – an initial £3.00 saving on antistatic clogs developed into a considerable loss when the new issue on contract had only 25% of the life of the previous style. Of course, user input could have the opposite effect, but conscientious, professional cooperation in selection can only enhance both the service to patients and the management of resources.

Management of resource materials not only involves the responsible approach to selection and purchasing, but also to storage and stock control. The rotation of stock is essential to ensure 'use by' dates are not over-run, and it has to be remembered that single use items cannot be re-sterilized even if unused (SHDD/DGH, 1989, HMSO 1984), e.g., a box of twelve sutures may result in a loss of between £8 and £150. Some individual products, like cardiac catheters and heart valves cost considerably more, over £400 each. Losses may also be incurred by incorrect storage causing damage, loss of sterile integrity, or in the case of drugs, deterioration.

Good management in clinical areas must also include the maintenance of adequate stock levels while avoiding excesses. Control of supplies must balance the current requirements with the risks incurred by overstocking – over-run of expiry dates, petty theft or improved models superceding current stock. The delegation of certain sections of stock control and management to selected staff can assist this important aspect of running an area as well as training staff in good practices.

Recent legislation (HMSO 1974) concerning consumer protection and product liability will not only have further effects on the choice of goods and materials, but also demand more rigorous control of stocks. The selection will require greater care to ensure products meet all current standards, and batching codes of items used on or in individual patients will have to be recorded in their notes. The effect of this new legislation is likely to be considerable, not only in increasing the costs of materials to ensure they meet the current standards, but also to assist users/consumers in recording batch coding. In addition more time will be required at the point of use to maintain the necessary documentation.

With advances in medical and technological knowledge the materials available will inevitably change and improve. The current views on atmospheric pollution may affect future materials used and methods of disposal. The users of the future will, no doubt, have to consider such aspects along with all the other factors.

9.4. Machinery and equipment

The selection and use of machines and equipment is in many ways similar to that of materials and sundries. However, this broad heading covers an ever-widening range of items used in patient care and treatment, e.g. ophthalmoscopes, heparin pumps, suction machines, operating tables and blood analysers, to name but a few. The questions of why, what, where and how, plus cost are again the most apt to commence the selection process. However, in many instances it is necessary to involve other professionals such as engineers, electricians, works officers or bacteriologists, as well as the users. Their help is invaluable in the initial stages, not only to ensure the acceptability of the equipment for installation and effective use, but also to provide a complete estimate of capital and revenue implications – the former must cover all aspects of installation including materials and manpower, while the revenue costs should account for all ongoing overheads, main supplies, materials and sundries required and maintenance, not to mention labour charges.

In addition all new equipment should meet with current British Standards and the requirements of the Health and Safety at Work etc. Act (1974). To ensure goods are acceptable in these respects, every item should be inspected by a suitably qualified professional person on delivery. It is a wise nurse manager who keeps a record of all items of machinery in her department, including information on purchase date, manufacturer and model details, and health and safety clearance. This, along with engineers' records can be invaluable in the future when making a case for replacements or providing information for legal purposes.

The purchase of equipment and machines normally falls into two categories, replacement of existing items and new machines. In either case it is essential to ensure funding is available to cover every aspect of purchase, installation and running costs including VAT.

Items such as beds and similar fundamental equipment are relatively simple to select, although variations of model or manufacture may obviously be preferable by virtue of suitability for the patients concerned or price. In other instances there may be only one supplier. Then careful enquiries are essential to ensure spare parts and servicing are readily available. Contact with established users can verify these issues, and give information on hidden costs or shortcomings.

In considering the purchase of replacement items thought must be given to existing practices, the availability of spare parts or accessories and maintenance arrangements. Many hospitals and health care units have a policy of standardization to simplify these issues and reduce costs. The full effects of deviation from such a practice must be carefully assessed, including those on patient care and possible treatment outcomes. Other problems can occur when simply replacing existing equipment with improved models, as the specification may have changed requiring considerable alteration to an existing procedure or management of the equipment itself – a change in the design of a resectoscope purchased as a replacement required the renewal of equipment used for sterilization. The cost was not outstanding but nevertheless it should have been included in the original estimates.

New equipment, especially that for new techniques, can have a considerable effect on the service, not only in the initial purchase but also on running costs. It has been shown that initially the number of patients treated is retained within that originally estimated and funded. However, as the users become more proficient and confident in the new apparatus and its results, the procedure time reduces, allowing an increase in the number of patients treated. This potential use must be accounted for in the pre-purchase estimate to ensure adequate revenue is available.

These revenue costs will be required to cover the running and maintenance of the equipment, including additional items or sundries to carry out the procedure. Examples are filters or tubing, power, access to and maintenance of a special environment for laser treatment. Without doubt there will be manpower implications, the extent depending on the breadth of skills, technology and clinical expertise required. Nevertheless these costs will make up a considerable proportion of the revenue costs.

New equipment in the first instance may also prolong operating lists or clinic sessions. While this might be accounted for during initial planning, adjustments will have to be made to overcome the effect on the work schedules of nursing and other support staff.

As experience and proficiency are gained it may be possible to treat more patients in the same allotted period of time. Care must be taken to anticipate the revenue implications in this instance as the man-hours may be similar but the additional 'per patient' costs overlooked.

Pitfalls abound for the unwary when accepting equipment as gifts. They may be VAT exempt, but has the installation cost been included, what are the revenue costs, and will the health board fund these in the long term? Past experience has demonstrated that it is essential to have detailed discussions with prospective benefactors, as it is often preferable to receive the funding to cover all aspects of the equipment rather than the actual item. In this way the users are able to select exactly what they require, can often use the Health Authority's/Board's negotiated preferential rates, but can still maintain the exemption from VAT. It also ensures that all aspects of installation and running costs are considered, especially for those machines or procedures which require a completely new team, however small.

The selection of machines and equipment can be compared to the purchase of a car or other large household item, and similar considerations must be accounted for prior to purchase – does the apparatus fulfil all the requirements of function, size, services, staffing, capital and revenue costs?

Like a car, will it start on demand? Is it comfortable enough? Will it fit into the garage? How convenient is it to be serviced, and are there competent mechanics to do this? Will the type of petrol required be available in the areas in which you travel? Finally, what is the cost, not only the purchase price, but the servicing costs, road tax and insurance?

9.4. Methods

As with all aspects of resource management, the 'method' by which any activity is undertaken will influence the outcome in every respect, including economy and effectiveness.

It is therefore essential that in establishing any procedure the objective is clearly identified at the outset. In this way, with careful planning, the most effective use of materials, machinery and man-power can be achieved, while maintaining a high standard of care. Reference to Chambers *Twentieth Century Dictionary* suggests that a 'method' is a system, technique, procedure, routine, model or plan. Each of these terms is well known in nursing parlance.

The majority of procedures are identified in the procedure book. The method or procedure for a sterile dressing, for example, will indicate the manpower requirements – one or perhaps two nurses and their grades, while the activities involved in dressing the wound will indicate the time factor, i.e., the man-hours. The trolley and suction apparatus are the machinery and equipment, well maintained and in good working order, while the lotions, dressing materials, suction catheter, strapping, disposal bag and nursing notes are the materials. However, additional and some-times forgotten factors are the time involved in explaining to the patient what is to happen before the trolley arrives, the hot water, soap and towels used to wash hands before and after the pro-cedure. Lastly account must be taken of portering and domestic services which might be involved in the disposal of refuse or similar associated tasks.

Methods or systems chosen to organize activities in other departments can equally have a significant effect on nursing and other groups. For example, a change in the admissions procedure for elective surgery from normal in-patient to day-patient care may increase the nursing workload on the day of surgery to include the admission procedure as well as pre- and post-operative care. In addition, the number of patients it will be possible to treat in one week will increase, further affecting nursing and other support service man-hours, either by the number, the shift pattern or both. Linen costs will increase along with those for theatre time, materials, machinery, service and manpower. Thus, while five-day wards can be more effective and efficient in the management of waiting lists, the use of some aspects of manpower, general services and bed usage, there will be no savings in materials, and other areas related to individual procedures or techniques in the clinical sense.

Similarly the treatment or technique chosen for certain patients' groups may alter the requirements of a ward or department sig-nificantly in all aspects of resources – as in urology where fibre optic equipment, advanced surgical and anaesthetic techniques, plus the arrival of the lithotrypter have changed the whole picture of treating renal calculi. In this instance nursing man-hours and bed occupancy per patient, with all the cost implications, have reduced, while the funding for machinery has risen markedly. Nevertheless, the outcome for the patients is earlier discharge, with improved results, minimal trauma and less discomfort.

9.6. Research

Research projects undertaken by different professional groups, but in particular the medical staff, are an ongoing activity in many hospitals. While most are funded from separate sources, e.g., Medical Research Council, pharmaceutical companies or special endowment funds, they can have implications on all resources to a greater or lesser degree.

The pre-approval costing for any research project should include the method, materials, manpower, machinery and the money or funding. The research funds or grant provided will cover most costs incurred during the prescribed period. However, problems can arise on completion of the project when the new procedure and all it involves is well established in a ward or clinic. Despite proving beneficial to the patient, unless NHS revenue is identified to continue the procedure or treatment, it should be discontinued. Anticipation of and a timely application to meet this need will prevent a situation known as 'creeping developments' – a cause of overspending – and the necessity to postpone the implementation of new procedures.

9.7. Money

Initially it was suggested that money is the single resource which affects every aspect of patient care. In the foregoing sections it has been mentioned frequently in relation to the purchasing and maintenance or support of materials, machinery, staffing and the method by which they are utilized. However, it is important to understand the way in which it is allocated and why, despite being government-funded, there are not only limits on the overall expenditure, but also for separate aspects of the service, e.g., capital projects, buildings, pharmacy, catering and domestic services.

9.7.1. Where does the money come from?

The National Health Service has to compete for its share of the government money against other departments like defence, housing and education. The allocation is therefore political and will vary according to which party is in government. In 1989 the funding was as follows.

1. General taxation 86%
2. National insurance 11%
3. Charges (prescriptions – dental – ophthalmic) 3%

However, this was augmented from donations and legacies commonly known as endowment funds.

9.7.2. Where does the money go?

Over 70% is spent on staff salaries, that is why the National Health Service is described as labour-intensive. The remaining 30% is spent on patient care and general services, e.g., drugs, medical equipment, food and servicing.

9.7.3. How is the money allocated?

Each November the spending for the current year is considered by the government. Money is allocated to Health Authorities in England and Wales according to national strategy known as RAWP (Resources Allocation Working Party) and in Scotland to Health Boards according to SHARE (Scottish Health Allocation Resource Equalization). Both strategies take into account the following factors.

1. The population covered by Health Authority/Board, i.e., number, age, sex, morbidity, mortality.
2. Existing services and number of staff employed.
3. Projected development, e.g., new buildings, staff training and expansion of preventative medicine.

A percentage for growth and development which includes inflation is added annually. Each Health Authority/Board has a statutory obligation to work within its budget. This can be very difficult and on occasions some drastic cutbacks are made so that they do not break the law.

9.7.4. How is spending controlled?

The money allocated to the Health Authorities/Boards is divided and allocated to the Districts (in England and Wales) and to the Units (in Scotland). There are different ways of allocating the money to hospitals and departments, and this can vary from one Health Authority/Board to another. However, once allocated to the hospital the funds are divided into what are called 'budgets'. A budget is therefore an allocation of money given to a budget-holder to provide a service for a period of time, usually one year. Budget-holders are normally heads of departments who are responsible for controlling staffing levels, ordering goods, providing services and maintaining their department's good order. Budget-holders have to know how much money they have to work with and how much of it has been spent at any given time, and therefore how much is still available. Therefore, at regular intervals, usually each month, the budget-holders receive a statement from the finance department. This is just like a bank statement although sometimes referred to as a 'fast form' and details all aspects of income and expenditure.

Historically budgets appear to have been designed according to tradition and practice, but under the new unit management structure budgets are now allocated for each area of care or unit. Unfortunately this presents the potential for a conflict of interests. Increasing emphasis is being placed on budget control, both at unit and ward/departmental level. In terms of the present financial position of the NHS all staff must be aware of departmental and ward financing, and how to encourage the economic use of hospital or clinic supplies and resources. A clinical budget represents the amount of money allocated to a particular ward or department for a year, the financial year of the National Health Service being from 1st April to 31st March.

It can be seen that the management of resources and finance in the NHS is difficult and complex, having to account for the existing services, changing and advancing technology and treatments, conflicting interests as well as demographic, public and political demands – virtually unlimited demands perhaps.

Computers and other forms of information technology have been commonplace in industry and commerce for many years. Health agencies, while perhaps not so advanced in this sphere, are increasingly using these programmes to assist in managing resources and nursing is no exception. The programmes will help in the forecasting of future workloads and resource requirements, the recording of usage and financial accounting. However, nurses will still require to use all their skills in personnel and resource management to maintain future staffing levels commensurate with high standards of care.

The management of resources could be likened to a child whose pocket money includes an allowance to cover the cost of feeding pet rabbits. A rise in the cost of food or an increase in the number of rabbits will cause the pocket money to be overspent. Controlling unplanned increases in the health service frequently seems like attempting to control reproduction in rabbits.

References

GMBATU (1985) *The Case Against Crown Immunity*, GMBATU, Hendon.

Guidance Document (1989) to the Consumer Protection Act (1987), *British Journal of Theatre Nursing*, 26, 5, pp 7–9.

HMSO (1974) *The Health and Safety at Work Act*, HMSO, London.

Lothian Health Board Sterilizing Centre (1988) *Comparative Cost Study of Disposable Hand Towels*, unpublished monograph.

Pearson, A. (1988) (Ed.) *Primary Nursing, Nursing in the Burford and Oxford Units*, Croom Helm Ltd, Beckenham.

Purdy, E., Wright, S., and Johnson, M. (1988) Change for the Better, *Nursing Times* 84, 38, pp 34–5.

Purdy, E., Wright, S., and Johnson, M. (1988) On the Right Track, *Nursing Times* 84, 39, pp 44–5.

Raybould, E. (1977) *A Guide for Nurse Managers*, Blackwood, London.

SHDD (1969) *Aberdeen Formula – Using Workload per Patient as a Basis for Staffing* SHS Studies No. 7.

SHDD/DGH (1989) The Re-use of Single-use Medical Devices *Sterile Supplies Information Letter* I p 74.

Telford, W.A. (1983) *Telford Method of Determining Nursing Establishments*, North Birmingham Health Authority, Sutton Coldfield.

Tiffney, T. (1984) The Marsden Experience, *Nursing Mirror* 159, 21, pp 28–30.

Further reading

Anthony, R.M. and Herzlinger, R. (1977) *Management and Control in Non-Profitmaking Organizations*, Irwin, USA.

Clay, T. (1987) *Nursing, Power and Politics*, Heinemann Nursing, London.

Stewart, R. (1963) *The Reality of Management*, Pan, London.

HMSO (1987) *The Consumer Protection Act*, HMSO, London.

HMSO (1989) *The Government Expenditure Plans*, C.M. 614, HMSO, London.

HMSO (1989b) *The NHS in Scotland – Looking for Patients*, HMSO, Edinburgh, London.

10

Research and information retrieval

Pauline Baber

10.1. Introduction to research (Why should I do it?)

'Research is done by other people!' This is a phrase echoed in many wards and departments by trained nurses who may have come into contact with nurse researchers as students. A number of nurse researchers, particularly educationists, use groups of student nurses in their work so it is quite possible that questionnaires have been completed, interviews given and some may even have been the subject of observations made by researchers whilst carrying out nursing duties.

During nurse training programmes there is often a research element in the Management of Care module, but it is likely that the students will have developed a research awareness of studies undertaken relevant to a particular aspect of health or disease rather than any feeling of compulsion to do a piece of research themselves.

With this background in mind it is not surprising that the statement at the beginning of this chapter is frequently made. But why should research be left to others? It is on the ward where questions are asked. For example, why are pressure areas cared for in a particular way; why is it necessary to fast a patient for a routine operation from 10 p.m. or 12 midnight the previous day when a patient for an emergency operation is considered safe for surgery after four to six hours fasting? Or why is it that when two patients of seemingly identical age, health and disposition have identical operations one appears to make a much quicker recovery than the other?

Research studies are done in order to effect change in nursing care and practice. The UKCC *Code of Professional Conduct* (1984) makes it clear in clauses three and ten that the registerd nurse, midwife or health visitor must maintain and improve professional knowledge and competence whilst having regard to the effects of the caring environment on the patient. Consideration of these clauses must lead the nurse to the importance of research, of the necessity to determine the answers to questions asked.

A well-known phrase from the *Report of the Committee on Nursing* (1972) reads, 'Nursing should become a research-based profession.' Some encouragement has been given to this concept during the past two or three decades by the award of fellowships for research projects and the development of university departments of nursing and nursing research units within universities, in addition to Open University courses on research and research workshops. However, as the above-quoted report states in paragraph 374, 'Direct research into clinical nursing . . . should begin in the ward itself . . . '

Who is to do this ward-based research? Some would say that there isn't time; there are too few nurses. If these attitudes prevail problems once uncovered will be submerged again, forgotten. Nursing will not advance because no change will be made, nor can be made until answers to identified problems have been sought and found.

The staff nurse is in an ideal position to identify problems and to seek by the research process to formulate answers. A staff nurse is often in a particular ward for a year or more, and once the ward, its routine and practices become familiar she will begin to ask, 'I wonder why . . . ?' or, 'Would it be better . . . ?' or, 'This piece of equipment seems to be causing problems, could it be improved?'

If support is needed for this statement that the staff nurse, or indeed any thinking nurse, should be undertaking research on the ward Evans (1980) provides abundantly in the following. He writes

The habits of mind which inform the everyday tasks of the nurse are exactly the same as those which undergird the very finest published research; in this way Everynurse ought not just to *do* simple research tasks as part of her work, but she ought also *always* to *be* a researcher, whether or not she writes or speaks a word in public. Nurses are given lots of token encouragement to participate in research or to be aware of the need for research-based nursing care, but not enough emphasis has been placed on those qualities of mind that essentially make the publishing scholar *identical,* in a way, to Everynurse, when she is truly being a nurse as she should. (Original italics.)

In addition to practical, ward-based research, a great deal of nurse education using research findings may take place in the ward environment. Whilst it has been said, and it is certainly true, that it is the ward sister who creates and maintains the learning climate of her ward (Orton, 1981) it is usually to the staff nurse the student nurse turns. She is seen as the person who knows the answers and yet a nurse, like themselves, directly involved in patient care. When problems are identified and the search for answers begins it must be seen as a good opportunity for teaching to take place. The staff nurse can teach students about recent advances in nursing and involve them in projects undertaken at ward level. This demands up-to-date knowledge of nursing research, and this can be achieved at a basic level by reading short articles on research in professional journals, with more in-depth study of research of particular interest to the reader.

Teaching can also be given in an upward direction by the staff nurse. She can make ward sisters, medical and paramedical staff aware of current nursing research, particularly if it involves patient care to the extent that a particular form of nursing care or treatment may not be the most beneficial to the patient, and that an alternative is available based on sound research principles. In this way she is helping to improve care for the patient in addition to doing her part in maintaining a good learning environment on the ward.

It will be seen from these introductory remarks that it is at the level of direct patient care that problems may be identified, and that answers may be sought. However, action needs to be taken.

10.2. Research methodology (How do I go about it?)

The following ideas for embarking on the research process in nursing are not intended to be an exhaustive account. It is realized that the reader will probably be planning her first piece of research, and the information given here will help her to begin. More detailed help may be gained from the suggestions for further reading at the end of the chapter, but the researcher learns most from actually doing a piece of research, particularly if it can be done with guidance from a more experienced researcher.

10.2.1. Seeking help

Some hospitals have a post of Research Advisor, or there may be a person in the college of nursing with research as part of their remit. Once a problem has been identified and a nurse feels that she would like to do some research she should make an appointment with the Research Advisor. Speaking with another person, especially a person who is able to guide on steps to be taken in the research process, will usually clarify the nurse's thoughts on the subject and crystallize the question to be asked.

Defining the question is the first step in the research process. One may have a hunch about something and the more thought that is given to the subject the stronger the hunch gets. However, the next step must be to see what is already written on the subject.

10.2.2. Literature search

The literature search should be carried out thoroughly no matter how small, or vague, the problem seems to be. It is always surprising to discover how many other people have had similar thoughts to oneself and have tackled a piece of research on the subject. Carrying out a literature search will reveal work done previously, if not on the actual subject, in related fields. Librarians in colleges of nursing often have a remarkable knowledge of the subject in question and can always give invaluable help in searching nursing bibliographies, obtaining articles and books from stock or from several other sources, and are also aware of others on the staff who may be doing work in similar areas and who may be able to give help.

Librarians have access to computerized bibliographies which can be of enormous help to the researcher. However, this should not be done early in the literature search. The researcher requires to have quite a lot of information on the subject in order to use computerized lists adequately. For example, one needs to be able to define key words in the problem. Key words cannot be identified until knowledge is considerable, and the researcher well on the way to defining the research question or constructing a hypothesis. If computerized bibliographies are used too soon many irrelevant references will be included, which not only waste time and cost money but may also lead the researcher away from her intended area of study.

10.2.3. Designing the study

Designing the study is an important part of research. What methods are to be employed? This is where the subject is important. Some research projects are descriptive studies, where the researcher makes an investigation of the characteristics of persons, objects or situations and the frequency with which certain phenomena occur, making an accurate portrayal of the relationships between them. Other research is supported by data produced by surveys using questionnaires, interviews and observations. Findings may lead the researcher to ask further questions, do more research and so be in a position to make recommendations for nursing practice.

10.2.4. Hypothesis

A hypothesis translates the research question into a statement of the predicted outcome of research on two, or more, variables. For example, in small-scale research done by the writer a hypothesis was constructed to state that 'The attitudes of student nurses towards caring for the elderly would become more positive as a result of education.'

10.2.5. Questionnaire: Construction and design

Many researchers feel that a questionnaire is essential to their enquiry. It is indeed a useful research tool but it is important to design it at the right time in the study and to design it well so that when it is used it gives the information desired by the researcher.

Some researchers begin their study by writing a questionnaire. This is inappropriate, because once the literature search has been done it is certain that the researcher's ideas will have changed as she has become more knowledgeable, and she will have the ability to formulate a much better questionnaire if she waits until she has acquired this knowledge.

Constructing a questionnaire can be difficult but the process may be assisted by the following information and hints, remembering that there is no such thing as the perfect questionnaire. However, the aim must be to make it as good as possible.

1. State the purpose of the enquiry, on a separate page before the questions begin.
2. Take care when constructing the items. Questions which may

appear to the researcher to be innocuous may cause hurt to others, or be ambiguous.
3. It is essential for the researcher to know what she is going to do with the information before obtaining it if the right questions are to be asked.
4. Anonymity of the respondents must be maintained, so develop a means of coding the questionnaires.

When the construction of a questionnaire is to be part of the research design one way of doing it is to jot down words, ideas, and opinions as the literature search progresses. After this it will be found that the basis of the questionnaire is already there. Care may then be taken in its construction to avoid the many pitfalls possible. Once constructed, ask another person to read the questionnaire. This can be very valuable especially if the person has knowledge and experience of research principles.

10.2.6. Seeking permission

It is necessary for permission to be obtained prior to carrying out research. As a general rule permission must be given if access to an institution to use its facilities or personnel is required, and initially, this may need to be at Health Board level. However, an approach to the principal nurse of the hospital will give information on sources of permission to be obtained, or the Research Advisor, if there is one, will be able to assist. Not only may the permission of the Health Board and principal nurse of the hospital be required, but if patients are to be involved Ethics Committees must be approached. Patients must also give their written permission and feel free to opt out. If the researcher wishes to involve student nurses she will require the permission of the Principal of the College of Nursing and Midwifery. One of the reasons is because students should not be over-exposed to nurse researchers who may desire their help in a number of different ways. If access to students is granted they, too, will be required to give written permission and to feel free to decline if they wish.

10.2.7. Pilot study

Consideration must now be given to a pilot study. A pilot study is a preliminary investigation useful in order to test a questionnaire or research tool, and to gain a measure of response from a small sample before embarking upon the main study. A pilot study should show up defects in a questionnaire in the form of ambiguity, items which probe too deeply and cause hurt, or questions which give information not required or conversely, do not give information which is required. A pilot study may also test the hypothesis by using a small part of the intended study; for example, by carrying out an investigation in one hospital when it is intended in the main study to use six hospitals. This small, preliminary study may give some indication of the outcome of the research, but may also serve to redirect the researcher along a different path if this should prove necessary.

10.2.8. Main study
The main study is the major part of the work. Consideration must be given to the dimensions of the study. For example, how many people is it going to involve? How many questionnaires? What will the cost be? I would reiterate the value of speaking to a person with research experience at the outset of the study. There is no point in embarking upon a study which is too large to be possible, or too small to be meaningful. If it is going to be expensive to send out questionnaires (and to pay for their return) it may be necessary to either limit the number or to choose different respondents to whom the researcher may have access with little cost. The advisor will be able to give invaluable help with the dimensions of the study, and to give ideas for sources of funding.

10.2.9. Analysing the results
The exciting part of undertaking research is obtaining the results. 'Is the study showing what I hope it will show?' 'Will the hypothesis be supported?' What the researcher chooses to do with the results depends, to some extent, on the reason for carrying out the research, and also the type of results obtained. In a small study all that may be needed in order to analyse the results is a pocket calculator. A study of moderate proportions, e.g., dealing with the responses to 80–100 items from up to 500 questionnaires may be analysed using a punch card developed by Copeland Chatterson (Cope-Chat Cards) by which data obtained may be sorted and stored manually. A computer is, of course, the ultimate method of storing data but if a computer is to be used advice on the most useful computer programs should be gained from a research statistician prior to commencing the study in order that only relevant data are collected. A research statistician will also be

able to advise on the significance of the results obtained, but if such a person is unobtainable considerable information on analysis of results and the methods available is contained in the suggestions for further reading.

10.2.10. Conclusion and implications

It follows logically from analysis of results that the researcher draws conclusions about the study. Has the hypothesis been supported? If it appears that the hypothesis has been supported to some extent it is probable that other research questions will have been raised and further work indicated. The reward of asking questions and actually doing a piece of research, is that it almost always leads the researcher to ask more questions and stimulates the desire to do further research.

10.2.11. Disseminating the results

Once conclusions have been made and the research as planned completed, it is necessary to write up the study and to tell others about it. The extent to which this is done depends on the stimulus for the study, its size and the findings. It is important, however, not to lose the value of the work done. The Research Advisor will again be able to assist on the most suitable method of disseminating the results, and to whom, indicating whether the research study should be published so that a wide audience may be informed of the work, or whether in the first instance it may be more appropriate to give a small, locally-based talk about it.

10.3. Summary (Has it been worth it?)

It is hoped that this short chapter will have given the reader sufficient knowledge and stimulus to be able to embark on a small research study. There is no doubt that the clinical areas contain much stimulus for research, and the staff nurse is in a good position not only to ask questions but to plan and implement a small study.

A research advisor will certainly ease the researcher's path by giving advice and encouragement throughout the process, but if such a person is unavailable this should not be a deterrent. Only experience will give the answer to the question, 'Has it been worth it?' but the experience gained during the process is invaluable, and even if the results are not earth-shattering the nurse should be stimulated to ask further questions, and she will surely find the research process easier next time.

References

Evans, D.L. (1980) Everynurse as Researcher: An argumentative critique of the principles and practice of nursing, *Nursing Forum*, 19, 4, pp 335–49.

HMSO (1972) *Report of the Committee on Nursing*, HMSO, London, paras 370, 374.

Orton, H. (1981) *Ward Learning Climate*, Royal College of Nursing, London, p 64.

UKCC (1984) *Code of Professional Conduct* (2nd Ed.), London.

Further reading

Chapman, M. and Mahon, B. (1986) *Plain Figures*, HMSO, London.

Cormack, D.F.S. (1984) (Ed.) *The Research Process in Nursing*, Blackwell Scientific Publications, Oxford.

Knapp, R.G. (1985) *Basic Statistics for Nurses* Wiley Medical, Chichester.

Polit, D.F., and Hungler, B.P. (1987) *Nursing Research: Principles and Methods* (3rd Ed.), Lippincott, Philadelphia.

Reid, N.G. and Boore, J.R.P. (1987) *Research Methods and Statistics in Health Care*, Edward Arnold, London.

Thomson, H. (1988) How to Understand Statistical Terms *Nursing Standard*, 3, 12, December 17.

Thomson, H. (1989) How to Present Data, *Nursing Standard*, 3, 30, April 22.

Wessex Regional Health Authority (1984) *The Research Process in Nursing: or, 'I wouldn't know where to Start!'* University of Southampton (videotape).

Index

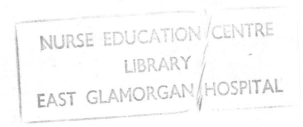